European Paedi Life Support Manual

Third Edition

Reprinted in July 2012

Reprinted in May 2014

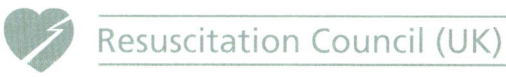

978-1-903812-27-3

European Paediatric Life Support Manual
Third Edition

Editors for Resuscitation Council (UK)

Ian Maconochie

Robert Bingham

Sarah Mitchell

Contributors

Souhail Alouni	Christine Fonteyne	Thomas Rajka
Dominique Biarent (ERC Course Director)	Miguel Felix	Sam Richmond
Paolo Biban	Mojca Groselj-Grenc	Antonio Rodriguez-Nunez
Robert Bingham	Sara Harris	Sheila Simpson
Keith Brownlee	Sylvia Hunyadi-Anticevic	Sophie Skellett
Gudrun Burda	Torsten Lauritsen	Frederic Tits
Gerard Cheron	Francis Leclerc	Felicity Todd
Fiona Clements	Anselmi Luciano	John Trounce
Karen Cooper	Jesus Lopez-Herce	Nigel Turner
Serena Cottrell	Ian Maconochie	Burkhard Wermter
Fotini Danou	David Mason	Mark Woolcock
Jo Draaisma	Sarah Mitchell	Jonathan Wyllie
Christoph Eich	Liz Norris	David Zideman

Originally published by the European Resuscitation Council (2003)

Second edition (2006)

Third edition (2011)

© Copyright: European Resuscitation Council and Resuscitation Council (UK)

This edition published by Resuscitation Council (UK) 2011
5th Floor, Tavistock House North, Tavistock Square, London WC1H 9HR
Tel: 020 7388 4678   Fax: 020 7383 0773   E-mail: enquiries@resus.org.uk   Website: http://www.resus.org.uk

Photographs © Mike Scott

ECGs © Oliver Meyer

Electrical conduction of the heart (Figure 8.6) © LifeART image (1989-2001) Wolters Kluwer Health, Inc.-Lippincott Williams & Wilkins. All rights reserved.

All rights reserved. No part of this publication may be reproduced or transmitted in any form or by any means, electronic, mechanical, photocopying, recording, or otherwise without the prior written permission of the Resuscitation Council (UK). Permission must also be obtained before any part of this publication is stored in any information storage or retrieval system of any nature.

Printed by: TT Litho Printers Limited
Corporation Street, Rochester, Kent. ME1 1NN
Tel: 01634 845397   Fax: 01634 846807   E-mail: admin@ttlitho.co.uk   Website: http://www.ttlitho.co.uk

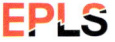

Foreword

The European Paediatric Life Support (EPLS) provider course is a pan-European project developed under the auspices of the European Resuscitation Council. It provides training for multidisciplinary healthcare professionals in the early recognition of the child in respiratory or circulatory failure and the development of the knowledge and core skills required to prevent further deterioration towards respiratory or cardiorespiratory.

The course comprises the manual, lectures, practical skill stations, teaching simulations and assessments. Candidate interaction and participation is a key element. This manual has been edited by members of the EPLS course Subcommittee of the Resuscitation Council (UK) for use in the UK.

Lectures

- Recognition of the seriously ill child
- Management of the seriously ill child
- Newborn resuscitation
- Post resuscitation care
- Ethics (group discussion)

Skill Stations

- Basic life support with BMV and choking
- Airway and ventilation
- Vascular access
- Arrhythmia recognition and safe defibrillation
- Trauma

Workshops

- Paediatric arrhythmias and management of cardiorespiratory arrest
- Trauma management

Teaching Simulations

- Respiratory failure
- Circulatory failure
- Trauma
- Cardiorespiratory arrest
- Newborn Resuscitation
- Cardiac arrhythmias

Instructors on the course teach voluntarily, giving their time and expertise without financial gain. Their enthusiasm and commitment for the subject helps to maintain the courses' high standards and ensure its availability to healthcare professionals who would be expected to apply the skills taught as part of their clinical duties.

We very much hope you enjoy the course.

Dr Ian Maconochie
Chairman, EPLS course Subcommittee,
Resuscitation Council (UK)

Sheila Simpson
Deputy Chairman, EPLS course Subcommittee,
Resuscitation Council (UK)

Glossary

- AED — Automated external defibrillator
- BLS — Basic life support
- BP — Blood pressure
- CRT — Capillary refill time
- CO_2 — Carbon dioxide
- CO — Cardiac output
- CPR — Cardiopulmonary resuscitation
- DNAR — Do not attempt resuscitation
- ECG — Electrocardiogram
- FiO_2 — Fraction of inspired oxygen
- HR — Heart rate
- IM — Intramuscular
- IO — Intraosseous
- IV — Intravenous
- Mg^{2+} — Magnesium
- O_2 — Oxygen
- PALS — Paediatric advanced life support
- PICU — Paediatric intensive care unit
- $PaCO_2$ — Partial pressure of arterial carbon dioxide
- PaO_2 — Partial pressure of arterial oxygen
- PEEP — Positive end expiratory pressure
- K^+ — Potassium
- RR — Respiratory rate
- SaO_2 — Arterial oxygen saturation
- SpO_2 — Peripheral oxygen saturation (pulse oximetry)
- SV — Stroke volume
- SVT — Supraventricular tachycardia
- SVR — Systemic vascular resistance
- VF — Ventricular fibrillation
- VT — Ventricular tachycardia

Throughout this publication the masculine is used to denote the masculine or the feminine

Contents

Chapter 1	Introduction to Paediatric Life Support	1
Chapter 2	Recognition and Initial Management of the Seriously Ill child	7
Chapter 3	Basic Life Support	17
Chapter 4	Advanced Management of the Airway and Ventilation	29
Chapter 5	Rhythm Recognition	43
Chapter 6	Emergency Circulatory Access, Fluid Administration and Medications	49
Chapter 7	Defibrillation and Cardioversion	59
Chapter 8	Management of Cardiorespiratory Arrest	65
Chapter 9	Principles of Post-resuscitation Care	75
Chapter 10	Special Situations in Paediatric Resuscitation	79
Chapter 11	The Injured Child	87
Chapter 12	Resuscitation of the Baby at Birth	101
Chapter 13	Ethical Considerations in Paediatric and Neonatal Life Support	113
Chapter 14	Human Factors and Quality in Resuscitation	117
Appendix 1	Paediatric Emergency Drug Chart	123
Appendix 2	Pulse Oximetry and Oxygen Therapy	125
Appendix 3	Asthma Algorithms	127
Appendix 4	Useful Websites	131

EUROPEAN PAEDIATRIC LIFE SUPPORT

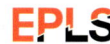

Introduction to Paediatric Life Support

CHAPTER 1

Learning outcomes

To understand:

- The aetiologies of cardiorespiratory arrest in children differ from those in adults
- The probable outcome of primary and secondary cardiorespiratory arrest
- Why specific anatomical and physiological properties of infants and young children influence their clinical management

Aetiologies of cardiorespiratory arrest

The aetiology of cardiorespiratory arrest in children differs from adults. This is due to anatomical, physiological and pathological differences which alter throughout childhood.

In adults, cardiorespiratory arrest is commonly due to a cardiac arrhythmia reflecting intrinsic heart disease. This **primary cardiorespiratory arrest** is an acute event and occurs without warning. Successful outcome is generally dependent on rapid defibrillation, as the most common arrhythmias encountered in primary cardiorespiratory arrest victims are ventricular fibrillation (VF) or pulseless ventricular tachycardia (VT). Every minute of delay until defibrillation results in the number of successful cases returning to spontaneous circulation decreasing by 10%.

In children, cardiorespiratory arrest is usually due to hypoxia, reflecting the limit of the body's ability to compensate for the effects of underlying illness or injury. Severe tissue hypoxia causes myocardial dysfunction, resulting in profound bradycardia which typically deteriorates to asystole or pulseless electrical activity (PEA). Both PEA and asystole are associated with a poor outcome.

This **secondary cardiorespiratory arrest** is rarely a sudden event, but a progressive deterioration. As respiratory and circulatory failure worsen (Figure 1.1), the body initially activates adaptive physiological responses aimed at limiting the effects of the deterioration on vital organs (compensated respiratory or circulatory failure). These adaptive responses will result in signs and symptoms that can be recognised, thereby providing an opportunity to intervene before further deterioration to cardiorespiratory arrest.

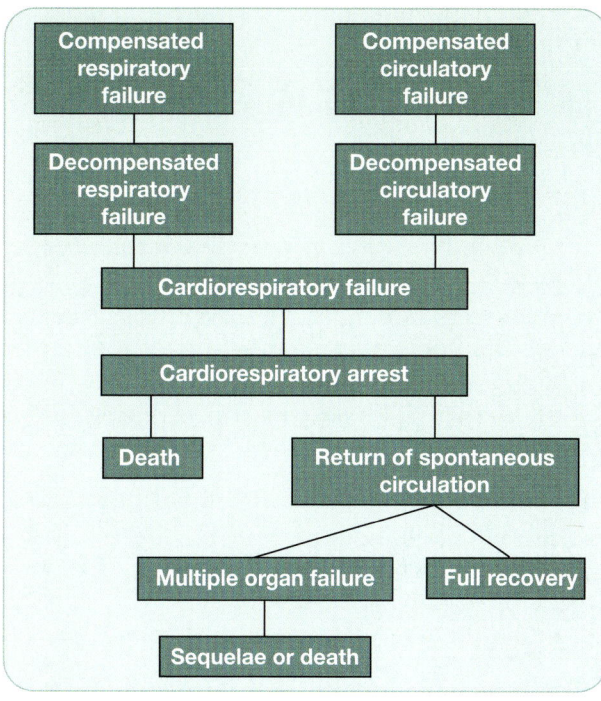

Figure 1.1 Consequences of progressive respiratory or circulatory failure

Outcome from secondary cardiorespiratory arrest

The outcome from secondary cardiorespiratory arrest is poor. Severe tissue hypoxia occurring before the heart stops means that all the vital organs are potentially seriously compromised; the heart finally arrests as a result of severe myocardial hypoxia.

Even if a return of spontaneous circulation (ROSC) is achieved, morbidity and mortality remains high. Many children succumb to severe organ injury (e.g. brain, kidney) or multi-system organ failure, 48-72 hours post arrest. Successful resuscitation from secondary cardiorespiratory arrest for out-of-hospital events is low (6-12% survival) and less than 5% of children will survive without neurological sequelae. In-hospital results are better (27% survival to discharge), but resuscitation from respiratory arrest, when there is still cardiac output, is associated with much better (50-70%) good quality, long-term survival.

Anatomical and physiological considerations

The underlying anatomical and physiological differences between infants, young children and adults largely account for the difference in aetiology of cardiorespiratory arrest.

The key differences will be considered in order of management priority based on the mnemonic ABCDE.

- A Airway
- B Breathing
- C Circulation
- D Disability (mental status)
- E Exposure

Airway

The infant/young child has an airway that is proportionately narrower and more susceptible to oedema and swelling than the adult. The absolute diameter of the airway is also smaller, and therefore respiratory infections account for a significantly higher level of morbidity and mortality in young children.

The effect of oedema and swelling can be seen in Poiseuille's law, which relates the resistance of the gas flowing through a tube (R) to its length (l), the viscosity of the gas (v) and the radius of the tube (r).

$$R = \frac{8l\,v}{\Pi\, r^4}$$

Thus a small decrease in the airway diameter has a huge effect on the flow of gases throughout the respiratory passages.

Relationship between head and neck

The infant's head is large in relation to the rest of their body. Since the occiput is protuberant, the head tends to flex on the neck when the infant is placed in a supine position. This leads to potential obstruction of the airway when the conscious level is reduced. With increasing age, the child's head becomes smaller in relation to their thorax, the neck lengthens and the larynx becomes more resistant to external pressure as tissues become less compliant.

Face and mouth

The infant's face is small and therefore the sizing of facemasks needs to be accurate otherwise it is difficult to achieve an effective seal. Additionally, pressure to the eyes can lead to damage and reflex bradycardia.

Inside the small mouth the tongue is relatively large. This combination means that airway obstruction is more likely in the unconscious infant/young child. The floor of the mouth is easily compressible; care is necessary to avoid compressing the soft tissues under the mandible to prevent airway obstruction when performing airway manoeuvres.

Nose and pharynx

The infant is a preferential nasal breather for the first six months or so of life. As a result, anything that causes nasal obstruction (e.g. anatomical abnormalities such as choanal atresia, copious secretions, nasogastric tubes or tapes) can lead to increased work of breathing and respiratory compromise.

The epiglottis in infants is larger and floppier than in adults. This means that it is vulnerable to damage by airway devices and manoeuvres.

The larynx

The larynx is higher in the infant compared to the older child and adult (where it is level with C5-6). Until about 8 years, the child's larynx is funnel shaped, with its narrowest segment at the level of the cricoid cartilage, as opposed to the olderchild/adult, who has a larynx that is cylindrical in shape. The anatomical variations have the following practical implications:

- Blind finger sweeps to remove a foreign body must not be performed in young children with partial airway obstruction as these may convert a partial into complete obstruction. The foreign body can become impacted into the narrowest part of the larynx (i.e. at the cricoid cartilage).

- The relatively large tongue may create airway obstruction as the epiglottis and larynx are higher in the neck.

- Control of the large tongue with a laryngoscope blade may be difficult.

- The high position of the larynx in a young child and infant creates a sharp angle between the oropharynx and the glottis. Direct visualisation of the glottis with the laryngoscope is therefore difficult. It may be easier to use a straight blade rather than a curved blade to obtain a view.

Breathing

Physiological considerations

The air-alveolar surface area for gas exchange in the lungs at birth is $3m^2$ compared with $70m^2$ in the adult. There is also a 10-fold increase in the number of small airways from birth to adulthood.

Normal respiratory function requires the movement of gas in and out of the lungs, and the exchange of oxygen (O_2) for carbon dioxide (CO_2) across the alveolar-capillary interface. Minute ventilation (the main determinant of CO_2 removal) depends upon the tidal volume (volume of gas with each breath) and the respiratory rate.

Spontaneous tidal volume stays constant throughout life at 6-8 ml kg^{-1}. It can be qualitatively assessed by auscultation of the chest, listening to air entry in the upper and lower zones of both sides of the chest.

Infants and small children have a relatively small resting lung volume and hence a low oxygen reserve. In addition, they have a high rate of oxygen consumption. This combination results in rapid falls in blood oxygen levels in respiratory compromise.

Mechanics of breathing

As they age, the mechanics of children's breathing changes. The infant has ribs that are cartilaginous and pliable, while their intercostal muscles are weak and relatively ineffective. The main muscle of respiration is the diaphragm. During inspiration, the diaphragm descends towards the abdomen, generating a negative pressure, which draws air into the upper airway and the lungs. Mechanical impedance to the contraction of the diaphragm (e.g. gastric distension, intestinal obstruction) will result in ineffective ventilation, as will any obstruction of the airway (e.g. bronchiolitis, asthma or foreign body aspiration).

In older children, the more developed intercostal muscles contribute significantly to the mechanics of breathing. The ribs ossify and act as a secure anchor for the muscles, as well as forming a more rigid structure that is less likely to collapse in respiratory distress. In children above 5 years the presence of significant intercostal recession should therefore be considered as an ominous sign and indicative of serious respiratory compromise.

Respiratory rate

Normal respiration requires minimal effort and the resting respiratory rate varies with age. The infant has a relatively high metabolic rate, oxygen consumption and carbon dioxide production, which is the main reason for their increased respiratory rates (Table 1.1). The respiratory rate also increases with agitation, anxiety and the presence of fever, therefore a record of respiratory rate as it changes over time is more useful than a single value.

Table 1.1 Respiratory rate ranges by age

Age (years)	Respiratory rate (breaths min^{-1})
< 1	30 – 40
1 – 2	26 – 34
2 – 5	24 – 30
5 – 12	20 – 24
> 12	12 – 20

Circulation and oxygen delivery

The circulating volume of the newborn is 80 ml kg^{-1} and decreases with age to 60-70 ml kg^{-1} in adulthood. This means that the total circulating volume of an infant is very small; e.g. 240 ml in a newborn of 3 kg and 480 ml in a 6 month old with a weight of 6 kg. Relatively small losses can be a significantly high percentage of their total circulating volume; this is why apparently minor diarrhoeal illnesses can result in considerable morbidity and even mortality in infants and young children.

Oxygen delivery (DO$_2$) to cells in the body's tissues is determined by arterial oxygen content and cardiac output. Arterial O$_2$ content (CaO$_2$) is determined by circulating haemoglobin, O$_2$ saturation plus the dissolved O$_2$ in the plasma.

Oxygen delivery to the body tissues

$$DO_2 = CaO_2 \times CO$$

DO$_2$ = oxygen delivery (ml min^{-1})
CaO$_2$ = arterial O$_2$ content (ml l^{-1})
CO = cardiac output (l min^{-1})

Arterial oxygen content

$$CaO_2 = Hb \times 1.34 \times SaO_2$$

Hb = haemoglobin concentration (g l^{-1}).

The constant 1.34 is the O$_2$ carrying capacity of 1 g of haemoglobin (ml O$_2$ g Hb^{-1}).

SaO$_2$ = oxygen saturation of haemoglobin (between 0 and 1 converted from percentage saturation value).

(SpO$_2$ is the peripheral oxygen saturation of blood which is, for practical purposes, almost identical to SaO$_2$).

If either of the parameters of DO$_2$ (CaO$_2$ and CO) decreases and is not compensated for by an increase in the other parameter, tissue O$_2$ delivery decreases.

In respiratory failure, the fall in CaO$_2$ can be compensated by increasing CO.

A decrease in CO, as in circulatory failure, cannot be compensated by a rise in O$_2$ content. It is accompanied immediately by a decrease in tissue O$_2$ delivery. It is also important to compare DO$_2$ with O$_2$ demand, which may be higher than normal (as in septic shock).

Heart rate

Stroke volume (i.e. the amount of blood ejected with each contraction of the heart) is relatively small in infancy (1.5 ml kg^{-1} at birth) and increases along with heart size. However, the cardiac output relative to body weight is higher than at any other stage of life (300 ml kg^{-1} min^{-1}, decreasing to 100 ml kg^{-1} min^{-1} in adolescence and 70-80 ml kg^{-1} min^{-1} in adults).

Cardiac output is the product of stroke volume and heart rate, and so the high cardiac outputs in infants and young children are primarily achieved by rapid heart rates (Table 1.2).

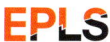

Chapter 1 Introduction to Paediatric Life Support

Table 1.2 Heart rate ranges (beats min⁻¹)

Age	Mean	Awake	Deep sleep
Newborn – 3 months	140	85 – 205	80 – 140
3 months – 2 years	130	100 – 180	75 – 160
2 – 10 years	80	60 – 140	60 – 90
> 10 years	75	60 – 100	50 – 90

Since cardiac output is directly related to the heart rate, bradycardia is a serious event and should be treated vigorously.

Systemic vascular resistance increases as the child ages and this is reflected in the changes seen in blood pressure ranges (Table 1.3).

Table 1.3 Blood pressure ranges by age

Age	Systolic blood pressure (mmHg)	
	Normal	Lower limit
0 – 1 month	> 60	50 – 60
1 – 12 months	80	70
1 – 10 years	90 + 2 x age in years	70 + 2 x age in years
> 10 years	120	90

Disability

The limited communication skills of infants and children have to be considered when attempting to assess neurological status. There is a tendency for ill children to regress to behaviour more befitting a younger child, especially if they are anxious or in pain. Effective pain control, empathy and appropriate language are therefore all essential factors when dealing with children. The presence of parents or other significant adults may help to alleviate many communication difficulties, as well as helping to allay fear and anxiety.

Conscious level is often determined by the Glasgow coma score and there is a modified scale for children under five years of age but a rapid assessment of the child's conscious level can be obtained by determining the AVPU score (Chapter 2). Additionally, assessment of pupil size and reaction, and the child's posture should be noted to determine neurological status.

Exposure

To ensure that no significant clinical information is missed, it is vital to examine the child fully by exposing their body. Appropriate measures to minimise heat loss (especially in infants) and respect dignity must be adopted at all times. The core body temperature should also be recorded and if necessary, appropriate measures to normalise it initiated.

Weight estimation

Medications are prescribed based on a child's body weight. In the emergency situation, it is often impractical to weigh them. It is therefore essential to have an alternative method of estimating weight as accurately as possible. Examples are the Broselow tape or the Sandell tape measure, which relates the length of the child to their body weight, or centile charts that estimate weight against age.

The following formula is commonly used to gain an approximate weight for children between 1-10 years:

$$(Age + 4) \times 2 = body\ weight\ (kg)$$

This formula is unsuitable for use in infants under 1 year. A term newborn infant averages a weight of 3.5 kg. By 6 months birth weight has normally doubled, and at 1 year trebled.

Although the actual weight of obese children will be underestimated by this formula, drug dosage is usually based on lean body mass, so it is still applicable. In addition, it's simplicity facilitates recollection under pressure.

Whatever method is used to establish the body weight of a child, it is essential that healthcare professionals are sufficiently familiar and competent in its use to be able to utilise it quickly and accurately.

Causes of death and prevention

In the neonatal period, the most common aetiology of death is congenital anomaly, followed by adverse perinatal events and sudden infant death syndrome.

In infancy, congenital anomaly is still the leading cause of death, followed by respiratory and cardiovascular illness, infectious disease and trauma.

The most common cause of mortality in pre-school children is trauma, followed by congenital anomaly, cardiovascular disease and malignancy. For school children, trauma is the major cause of death, with half as many deaths again caused by malignancy.

Accident prevention schemes need to be tailored to the different age groups. Such schemes depend on a combination of three elements: education, alteration of environmental hazards and the enforcement of safety legislation. All healthcare professionals should be involved in injury prevention:

- Primary prevention (prevention of the accident) e.g. by using safe material in playgrounds

- Secondary prevention (reducing the effects of an accident) e.g. by promoting the wearing of bicycle helmets

EUROPEAN PAEDIATRIC LIFE SUPPORT

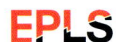

- Tertiary prevention (diminishing the consequence of the event by improving the effectiveness of emergency services after injury) e.g. taking part in a structured course such as EPLS

Expected and unexpected death

The death of a child is emotionally distressing for parents, relatives and the healthcare professionals involved. This latter group may include pre-hospital staff as well as those based at the hospital. An opportunity to hold a debriefing session for all staff after the death is important to allow them to air any concerns, feelings or emotions that arise from having delivered care to the child. Any member of the healthcare team should feel able to seek help and advice, from colleagues, their general practitioner (GP), bereavement counsellors or occupational health if they feel they require it.

There are two interrelated processes for reviewing child deaths in the UK since April 2008: a rapid response by a group of key professionals who come together for the purpose of enquiring into and evaluating each unexpected death of a child and an overview of all child deaths (under 18 years) undertaken by child death overview panels (CDOPs), who report to the local safeguarding children's board (LSCB) of each area.

The GP, health visitor (for children under 5 years) and school nurse (for children over 5 years) must be informed about any paediatric deaths. In the UK, it is common practice to invite the parents approximately 4-6 weeks after the child's death to meet with the consultant in charge. This enables the parents to ask any questions and to receive information about the results of investigations that have taken place. The consultant would usually also be available to answer questions arising about the care that the child received.

A child may have a condition for which it is agreed that resuscitation would not be beneficial. Looking after such a child and his family requires compassionate and considered management (palliative care) and is beyond the scope of the EPLS course.

It is important to feel that the best possible care has been delivered as not all resuscitation attempts are successful. Early intervention based on the ABCDE approach will reduce the number of unexpected deaths. The EPLS course aims to provide this structured approach for the optimal care of children.

Key learning points

- The respiratory and circulatory anatomy and physiology of infants and young children influence both the aetiology and the management of their illnesses/injuries
- Children are more likely to suffer a secondary, rather than a primary cardiorespiratory arrest
- Successful resuscitation from respiratory arrest, where there is still a cardiac output, is associated with 50-70% good quality, long-term survival
- Survival from full secondary cardiorespiratory arrest without neurological sequelae is considerably less likely (< 5% out of hospital and approximately 27% in hospital)
- The mnemonic ABCDE is the basis of both the assessment and the management of seriously ill/injured children

Further reading

Atkins DL, Everson-Stewart S, Sears GK, Daya M, Osmond MH, Warden CR, Berg RA; Resuscitation Outcomes Consortium Investigators. Epidemiology and outcomes from out-of-hospital cardiac arrest in children: the Resuscitation Outcomes Consortium Epistry-Cardiac Arrest. Circulation 2009; 24;119:1484-91.

Berg MD, Nadkarni VM, Berg RA. Cardioplumonary Resuscitation in Children. Curr Opin Crit Care. 2008;14:254-60.

Deasy C, Bernard SA, Cameron P et al. Epidemiology of paediatric out-of-hospital cardiac arrest in Melbourne, Resuscitation 2010; 81: 1095-1100.

Donoghue AJ, Nadkarni V, Berg RA, Osmond MH, Wells G, Nesbitt L, Stiell IG. Out-of-Hospital Pediatric Cardiac Arrest: An Epidemiologic Review and Assessment of Current Knowledge Ann Emerg Med. 2005;46:512-522.

Dudley NC, Hansen KW, Furnival RA, Donaldson AE, Van Wagenen KL, Scaife ER. The effect of family presence on the efficiency of pediatric trauma resuscitation. Ann Emerg Med 2009; 53: 777-784, e3.

Lopez-Herce J, Garcia C, Rodriguez-Nunez A, Dominguez P, Carillo A, Calvo C, Delgado MA. Long term outcome of paediatric cardiorespiratory arrest in Spain. Resuscitation 2005: 64:79-85.

Nadkarni VM, Larkin GL, Peberdy MA, Carey SM, Kaye W, Mancini ME, et al. First documented rhythm and clinical outcome from in-hospital cardiac arrest among children and adults. JAMA. 2006; 4;295:50-7.

Tibballs J, Kinney S. A prospective study of outcome of in-patient paediatric cardiopulmonary arrest. Resuscitation 2006;71;310-8.

Topjian AA, Nadkarni VM, Berg RA. Cardiopulmonary resuscitation in children. Curr Opin Crit Care. 2009; 15:203-8.

Website: The Children's Action Prevention Trust www.capt.org.uk

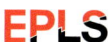

Recognition and Initial Management of the Seriously Ill child

CHAPTER 2

> ## Learning outcomes
>
> To understand:
> - The importance of early recognition of the seriously ill child
> - The importance of the structured ABCDE approach to rapidly identify potential respiratory, circulatory and/or central neurological failure in the seriously ill child
> - The importance of the structured ABCDE approach to prioritise and assess effectiveness of initial management strategies

Early recognition of the seriously ill child

In children, cardiorespiratory arrest is usually due to hypoxia, reflecting the end of the body's ability to compensate for the effects of underlying illness or injury. The initial problem may originate from the airway, breathing or circulation. Irrespective of the primary aetiology, cardiorespiratory arrest in children is rarely a sudden event, but a progressive deterioration from combined respiratory and circulatory failure.

Early recognition and effective management of respiratory and/or circulatory failure will prevent the majority of paediatric cardiorespiratory arrests and thus reduce morbidity and mortality. It can also help identify children for whom cardiorespiratory resuscitation may be inappropriate which can help facilitate suitable palliative care.

The principles outlined in this chapter apply to the seriously ill child in all environments, i.e. the acute hospital setting or out-of-hospital. Use of the structured ABCDE approach (detailed later in this chapter) helps to ensure that potentially life-threatening problems are identified and managed in order of their priority.

A: Airway problems

A review of practical airway management procedures is provided in Chapter 4.

Causes of airway obstruction

Airway obstruction can be partial or complete, sudden or insidious, progressive or recurrent. Respiratory rate and work of breathing generally increase in airway obstruction. When assessing airway patency, **chest movement does not guarantee that the airway is clear.** Air entry needs to be assessed as well by looking, listening and feeling for air movement, and by chest auscultation.

Initially, airway obstruction is often partial but can lead to respiratory failure, exhaustion, secondary apnoea and eventually hypoxic brain damage. Additionally, partial airway obstruction can rapidly become total, and result in cardiorespiratory arrest.

Congenital abnormalities such as choanal atresia or Pierre-Robin syndrome can be initially managed by use of an appropriate airway adjunct to open the airway and buy time, prior to definitive treatment.

Depression of the central nervous system can cause loss of airway control as protective upper airway reflexes are lost. This may be compounded in the infant due to the age related anatomical features. The pronounced occiput and short neck causes head flexion in the supine position and, together with the proportionately large tongue, can quickly lead to airway obstruction in the unconscious infant.

Causes of central nervous system depression include head trauma, metabolic disorders (e.g. hypoglycaemia, inborn errors of metabolism), hypercapnia, alcohol and medications (e.g. opiates, benzodiazepines). Airway obstruction due to these causes may not be accompanied by tachypnoea or increased work of breathing.

> ### Table 2.1 Causes of airway obstruction
>
> - Congenital abnormality (e.g. choanal atresia, Pierre-Robin syndrome)
> - Secretions (e.g. vomit, blood)
> - Respiratory tract infections (swelling or mucus secretions)
> - Nasal feeding tubes
> - Oxygen delivery devices (e.g. nasal cannulae)
> - Foreign body (e.g. food, toy, orthodontic appliances)
> - Central nervous system depression (loss of muscle tone)
> - Pharyngeal swelling (e.g. oedema, infection)
> - Epiglottitis
> - Laryngotracheobronchitis (croup)
> - Trauma (facial or throat)

Recognition of airway obstruction

Airway obstruction may be demonstrated by difficulty in breathing and/or increased respiratory effort. In a conscious child there may be visible distress. There may be additional respiratory noises, such as inspiratory stridor, if the obstruction is partial. Causes are seen in Table 2.1.

EUROPEAN PAEDIATRIC LIFE SUPPORT

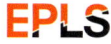

Management of airway obstruction

The treatment of partial airway obstruction is to maintain airway patency and ensure that it does not become totally occluded. This may be achieved by head positioning, clearance of any secretions or foreign bodies, and summoning further assistance as indicated.

In patients with airway obstruction, delivery of supplemental oxygen is advised as early as possible, to minimise the potential effects of hypoxia.

The conscious child will usually adopt a position that optimises airway patency. If the child is stable, and deterioration is considered unlikely, he should be left with his parents/carers who can help administer oxygen and minimise stress and anxiety. Feeding should be avoided, and any fever treated to reduce increased metabolic demand. If there is a decreased level of consciousness, airway compromise must be assumed. The management priorities are to get more help whilst safeguarding the airway and preventing complications such as aspiration of gastric contents, by placing the child in the recovery position or supporting the head-up position.

Basic airway opening manoeuvres (e.g. head tilt and chin lift or jaw thrust) should be used. Adjuncts such as oro/nasopharyngeal airways can also be used until more experienced help is available. Advanced emergency airway management may involve insertion of a tracheal tube, laryngeal mask airway (LMA) or cricothyroidotomy, although the latter will only provide temporary oxygenation until a definitive airway can be achieved.

B: Breathing problems

In all seriously ill or injured children, the priority is for the appropriate management of the airway and ventilation (breathing).

Causes of breathing (respiratory) problems

Respiratory failure can result from acute or chronic breathing inadequacy. Movement of air into and out of the lungs (ventilation) and/or gas exchange at the alveolar capillary interface may be compromised. The underlying problem may be due to lung pathology (i.e. congenital or acquired diseases or trauma) or have a non-respiratory origin (e.g. circulatory failure, metabolic disorder, neurological problem).

Failure of ventilation results in CO_2 accumulation. Oxygen levels also fall but this can be corrected by raising the inspired oxygen fraction. Failure of gas exchange across the alveolar-capillary interface is often a result of fluid accumulation within the alveoli (pulmonary oedema or infection) and results in a fall in arterial O_2 levels and increased lung stiffness, i.e. decreased lung compliance. Other common causes of the failure of gas exchange include bronchospasm and atelectasis, which are also associated with stiff lungs. The arterial O_2 levels fall, which stimulate breathing via peripheral chemoreceptors (the aortic and carotid bodies).

Arterial CO_2 levels may initially be normal or even low although they will rise, stimulating the respiratory centre to increase the respiratory rate, as failure worsens. The work of breathing then increases not only due to the increased respiratory rate but also due to the increased lung stiffness.

Increased arterial CO_2 levels may also result in tachycardia, vasodilatation and bounding pulses, but these are unreliable findings.

The respiratory rate can be classified as abnormal if it is too rapid (tachypnoea), too slow (bradypnoea) or absent (apnoea). Respiratory distress is a clinical syndrome which reflects increased work of breathing, often associated with attempts to increase tidal volume and can be associated with either tachypnoea or bradypnoea.

As the work of breathing increases, an increased proportion of the cardiac output is diverted to the respiratory muscles with a consequent increase in the amount of carbon dioxide produced.

Ultimately, if the respiratory system is unable to provide sufficient oxygen for tissue requirements, anaerobic metabolism occurs and respiratory acidosis is complicated by metabolic acidosis.

Recognition of respiratory failure

From a physiological viewpoint, respiratory failure is usually defined as failure of the respiratory system to maintain an arterial oxygen level (PaO_2) > 9 kPa with 21% inspired O_2 (air) or/and arterial carbon dioxide level of ($PaCO_2$) < 6.5 kPa. This definition requires arterial blood gas analysis, which can be difficult to obtain and is unreliable in children. However, a PaO_2 of 9 kPa corresponds approximately to a peripheral oxygen saturation (SpO_2) of 90%.

A child with respiratory distress may be able to maintain their arterial blood gases values within relatively normal limits by increasing their respiratory effort. It is therefore important to evaluate whether the child's situation is stable or if decompensation to respiratory failure is imminent. This evaluation requires knowledge of the signs and symptoms of respiratory distress and/or respiratory failure. When the compensatory mechanisms fail, deterioration is rapid and imminent cardiorespiratory arrest must be anticipated.

Warning signs are:

- Decreased level of consciousness
- Hypotonia
- Decreased respiratory effort
- Cyanosis or extreme pallor (despite oxygen being given)
- Sweating
- Bradycardia

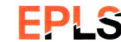

In children, recognition of respiratory failure is based on the full assessment of respiratory effort and efficacy, and the identification of evidence of respiratory inadequacy on major organs.

Work of breathing

Evidence of increased work of breathing is based on observation of the following:

- Increased respiratory rate
- Intercostal recession
- Sternal recession
- Subcostal recession
- Use of accessory muscles (e.g. nasal flaring)
- Head bobbing

Respiratory rate

Tachypnoea is frequently the first indication of respiratory insufficiency. Normal respiratory rates vary with age and this must be considered when determining the presence of tachypnoea (Table 2.2).

Table 2.2 Respiratory rate ranges by age	
Age (years)	Respiratory rate (breaths min^{-1})
< 1	30 – 40
1 – 2	26 – 34
2 – 5	24 – 30
5 – 12	20 – 24
> 12	12 – 20

Changes in respiratory rate over time are very important. An increasing respiratory rate represents increasing physiological compensation against the deterioration in respiratory function. A sudden reduction in the respiratory rate in an acutely ill child is an ominous sign and may be a pre-terminal event. Causes may include exhaustion, central nervous system depression or hypothermia. Fatigue is always an important consideration in children: an infant with a respiratory rate of 80 min^{-1} will tire quickly.

Recession

Recession (or retractions) may be sternal, subcostal or intercostal. The degree of recession gives an indication of the severity of respiratory disorder. Infants and young children can exhibit significant recession with relatively mild to moderate respiratory compromise, owing to their highly compliant chest wall. However, in children over approximately 5 years (by which age the chest wall is less compliant) recession is a sign of significant respiratory compromise.

Use of accessory muscles

When the work of breathing is increased, the sternocleidomastoid muscles in the neck are often used as accessory respiratory muscles. In infants, this may cause the head to bob up and down with each breath. This 'head bobbing' actually reduces the efficiency of each breath.

'See-saw' respiration

A breathing pattern, described as 'see-saw' respiration, is sometimes observed in severe respiratory compromise. It is the paradoxical movement of the abdomen during inspiration, i.e. the abdomen expands and the thorax retracts as the diaphragm contracts. This is inefficient respiration because the tidal volume is reduced, despite the increased muscular effort.

Inspiratory and expiratory noises

Normally, the airway above the thoracic inlet (extrathoracic) narrows and the airway below (intrathoracic) widens during the inspiratory phase of breathing. This pattern reverses on expiration. Observing the timing of an abnormal noise can indicate the site of airway obstruction. The presence of a high-pitched inspiratory noise (stridor) is characteristic of an upper airway (extrathoracic) obstruction and is due to rapid, turbulent flow through a narrowed portion of the upper tracheal airway. In severe obstruction, the stridor may also occur on expiration (biphasic stridor) but is usually less pronounced than it is during inspiration.

Wheezing is generally an expiratory noise. It is indicative of lower (intrathoracic) airway narrowing, usually at bronchiolar level, and may be audible with the ear, or only on chest auscultation with a stethoscope.

The volume of airway noises is not indicative of the severity of respiratory compromise; diminishing noises may be indicative of increasing airway obstruction or exhaustion of the child.

Grunting

Grunting is mainly heard in neonates and small infants, but can also occur in young children. It is the result of exhaling against a partially closed glottis, and is an attempt to generate a positive end-expiratory pressure thus preventing airway collapse at the end of expiration. Grunting is generally associated with 'stiff' lungs (e.g. respiratory distress syndrome, pulmonary oedema, atelectasis). Regardless of the underlying condition, grunting is an indication of severe respiratory compromise.

Nostril flaring

Flaring of the nostrils is often seen in infants and young children with increased respiratory effort.

Position

Children in respiratory distress will usually adopt a position to maximise their respiratory capacity. In upper airway obstruction, they often adopt a 'sniffing the morning air' position to optimise their upper airway patency. In generalised or lower respiratory problems, children often sit forward, supporting their weight on their arms, and holding on to (or wrap their arms around) their knees. This position results in a degree of shoulder girdle 'splinting', which enhances accessory muscle use. The child should be supported in the position of optimal airway maximisation/comfort for them and have oxygen therapy given accordingly.

The degree of respiratory distress generally provides clinical evidence of the severity of respiratory insufficiency. However, there are three general exceptions to this (Table 2.3).

Table 2.3 Exceptions to increased work of breathing in respiratory failure

1. Exhaustion – children who have had severe respiratory compromise for some time may have progressed to decompensation and no longer show signs of increased work of breathing

   Exhaustion is a pre-terminal event

2. Neuromuscular diseases (e.g. muscular dystrophy)

3. Central respiratory depression – reduced respiratory drive results in respiratory inadequacy (e.g. encephalopathy, medications such as morphine)

Efficacy of breathing

The infant's relatively higher metabolic rate and oxygen consumption accounts for their increased respiratory rates (Table 2.2). Thus the effectiveness of breathing can be assessed by respiratory rate together with tidal volume, which in turn is evaluated by observation of chest movement, palpation, auscultation and percussion. Additional information can be easily obtained by non-invasive pulse oximetry.

Chest movement, palpation and percussion

Observation of chest movement demonstrates the extent and symmetry of chest expansion. As well as revealing increased work of breathing, observing the movement of the chest wall can help identify diminished or asymmetrical respiratory effort.

Palpation of the chest wall may identify deformities, surgical emphysema or crepitus.

Percussion of the chest wall can demonstrate areas of collapse (dullness) or hyper-resonance (e.g. in pneumothorax).

Chest auscultation

When listening with a stethoscope, air entry should be heard in all areas of the lungs. Volume of air movement occurring with inspiration and expiration can be estimated by auscultation. It is useful to compare the areas on one side of the chest with the other.

A very quiet or near silent chest indicates a dangerously reduced tidal volume and is an ominous sign.

Pulse oximetry

A pulse oximeter should be used on any child with potential respiratory failure. An arterial oxygen saturation (SpO_2) of < 90% in air or < 95% in supplemental oxygen indicates respiratory failure.

It should be noted that SpO_2 measurements are unreliable when a child has a poor peripheral circulation, carboxyhaemoglobin or methaemoglobin. When SpO_2 is < 70% pulse oximetry is inaccurate, although trends will still be reliable.

Central cyanosis appears when the SpO_2 level is < 80% (it indicates that desaturated haemoglobin is > 5 g dl^{-1}). The absence of cyanosis, particularly in anaemic patients, does not imply that the blood oxygen levels are normal. Cyanosis is an inconsistent sign of respiratory failure. It is most apparent on the mucosae of the mouth and in the nail beds. Cyanosis limited to the extremities is usually due to circulatory failure (peripheral cyanosis) rather than to respiratory failure (central cyanosis). Hypoxia may also cause vasoconstriction and skin pallor, which will mask cyanosis. However, in a child with acute respiratory compromise, the development of central cyanosis is a late indication of severe hypoxia and **is a pre-terminal sign.**

Effects of respiratory inadequacy on other body organs

Ongoing respiratory compromise rapidly affects other body organs/systems.

Heart rate

Hypoxia initially causes tachycardia. As this is a non-specific sign it needs to be considered alongside other clinical signs. Severe or prolonged hypoxia ultimately leads to bradycardia and therefore it is important to observe for trends rather than absolute values in heart rate. In a severely hypoxic child, **bradycardia is a pre-terminal sign.**

Skin perfusion

Hypoxia produces vasoconstriction and pallor of the skin. As their clinical condition deteriorates, the child's colour may become mottled before cyanosis appears centrally (lips and mouth).

Conscious level

Hypoxia and/or hypercapnia initially lead to agitation and/or drowsiness. Ongoing cerebral hypoxia ultimately results in loss of consciousness. In infants and young children, initial cerebral hypoxia may be difficult to detect but their parents/carers frequently report that the baby/child is not responding to them as usual. This information is important and should not be ignored. The level of consciousness should be assessed using the AVPU score (Table 2.4).

Generalised hypotonia also accompanies cerebral hypoxia.

EUROPEAN PAEDIATRIC LIFE SUPPORT

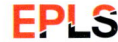

Table 2.4 The level of consciousness

- **A** ALERT
- **V** responds to VOICE
- **P** responds to PAIN
- **U** UNRESPONSIVE to painful stimuli

The management of respiratory compromise

The treatment of breathing problems is dependent on achieving a patent airway and effective delivery of oxygen. The method of oxygen administration will vary according to the child's clinical condition and age. Children who have adequate spontaneous breathing should have high-flow oxygen delivered in a manner that is non-threatening (when agitated the child's airflow will become turbulent and resistance to flow will increase) and best tolerated by them, e.g. from a free-flow device held by their parents, a non-rebreathing facemask or nasal cannulae.

When breathing is inadequate (or absent) high-flow oxygen should be delivered by ventilation with a bag and mask system. In situations where the child is exhausted and is likely to need ongoing respiratory support, tracheal intubation may be indicated.

C: Circulatory problems

The appropriate management of the airway and ventilation (breathing) is the priority in all seriously ill children and should be addressed before considering their circulatory status.

Circulatory failure and shock

Shock is a clinical state where the delivery of oxygenated blood (and associated delivery of nutrients e.g. glucose) to the body tissues is inadequate for metabolic demand. Additionally, the removal of cellular waste (e.g. CO_2, lactic acid) may also be impaired. Circulatory failure refers to insufficient blood being delivered to the body's tissues.

Shock may occur with increased, normal or decreased cardiac output (CO) or blood pressure (BP). Initially, the child's body can physiologically compensate for reduced tissue perfusion. However, when blood pressure starts to fall, as seen in circulatory failure, perfusion of the vital organs (e.g. brain, myocardium, kidneys) becomes increasingly compromised. Inadequate tissue blood flow results in anaerobic metabolism and lactic acid accumulation occurs. The resultant cell damage may be irreversible. It is therefore very important to promptly recognise and treat any child with compensated circulatory failure, to prevent deterioration to a decompensated state.

Compensated circulatory failure may have a normal blood pressure, but signs of abnormal perfusion, tachycardia, poor skin perfusion, weak peripheral pulse, tachypnoea and oliguria are observed.

Decompensated circulatory failure is present when hypotension develops and vital organ perfusion is compromised. The clinical signs of inadequate tissue perfusion are much more apparent.

Aetiology of shock

Shock can arise from circulatory or respiratory failure. Most children with sustained shock, whatever its aetiology, have some degree of cardiovascular dysfunction requiring more than one type of treatment (i.e. managing the airway, breathing and circulation).

Although CO is usually decreased in circulatory failure, septic and anaphylactic shock may be characterised by high CO. In this case, the systemic vascular resistance (SVR) is low and the child seems to be well perfused with bounding peripheral pulses and an increased pulse pressure (the difference between the systolic and diastolic BP). Even in the presence of increased CO and apparently good perfusion, the metabolic requirements are not fulfilled owing to mismatch between blood flow and tissue demand.

The most common causes of circulatory failure in children are hypovolaemia, sepsis or anaphylaxis.

Hypovolaemic shock: Characterised by decreased circulating volume (preload). It may result from severe fluid loss (as in dehydration) or haemorrhage.

Distributive shock: Typified by inadequate distribution of blood, so that the blood flow is insufficient for the metabolic demand of the tissues (e.g. anaphylaxis, sepsis or neurogenic).

Cardiogenic shock: Circulatory failure is less commonly the result of a primary cardiac problem due to congenital or acquired heart disease (e.g. cardiomyopathy, myocarditis or following cardiac surgery).

Obstructive shock: An uncommon cause of circulatory failure due to obstruction of blood flow to/from the heart (e.g. tension pneumothorax, cardiac tamponade or constrictive pericarditis).

Dissociative shock: Characterised by insufficient oxygen carrying capacity of the blood (e.g. anaemia or carbon monoxide poisoning).

Evaluation of the circulatory system

Oxygen delivery to the tissues is dependent on the arterial oxygen content and the CO. The CO is the product of the blood volume ejected from the left ventricle with each contraction and the heart rate.

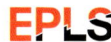

> **Cardiac output**
> **CO = HR x SV**
> CO = cardiac output.
> HR = heart rate.
> SV (stroke volume) = blood volume ejected with each contraction.

> **Blood pressure**
> **BP = CO x SVR**
> BP = blood pressure.
> SVR = systemic vascular resistance.

Of the variables affecting or affected by cardiac output (Figure 2.1), some can be easily measured (HR and BP) and others (SV and SVR) must be indirectly assessed by examining the amplitude and quality of pulses, and the adequacy of end-organ perfusion (mental status, capillary refill time, skin temperature and, when available, urine output).

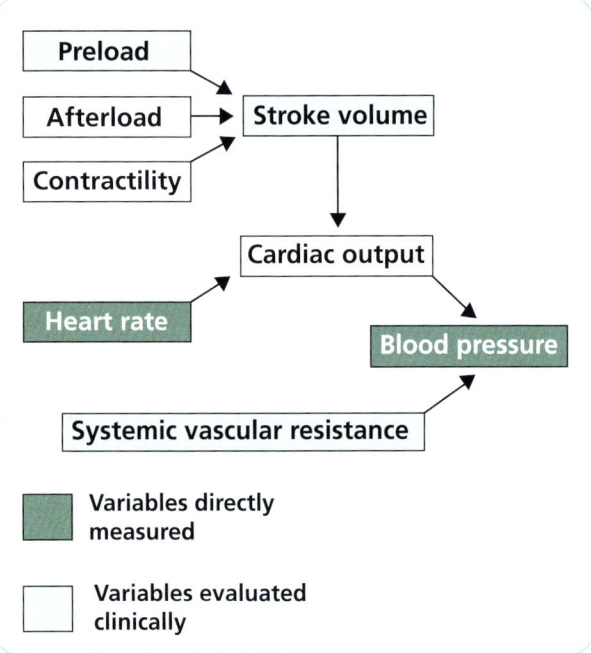

Figure 2.1 Evaluation of cardiovascular relationships

A low SVR or CO can be suspected if the systolic BP is below the normal range for the child's age.

Recognition of circulatory failure

In children, the recognition of circulatory failure is based on a complete cardiovascular assessment, looking for the effects of any circulatory insufficiency on major organs.

Parameters evaluated include:

- Heart rate
- Pulse volume
- Capillary refill time
- Blood pressure
- End organ perfusion status

Heart rate

The heart rate initially rises to maintain cardiac output.

Sinus tachycardia is a common response to many situations, e.g. pain, anxiety, fever but it is also seen in hypoxia, hypercapnia and hypovolaemia. When tachycardia is accompanied by other signs of circulatory insufficiency, it is evidence of the body's attempts at physiological compensation. Neonates have limited cardiac reserve; they increase their CO primarily by increasing heart rate rather than stroke volume (SV). They develop bradycardia as the first response to hypoxia unlike older children.

When the increased heart rate is unable to maintain adequate tissue perfusion, the tissue hypoxia and acidosis result in bradycardia. **The presence of bradycardia is a pre-terminal sign**, indicating that cardiorespiratory arrest is imminent.

Pulse volume

Feeling for the volume (or amplitude) of central pulses (e.g. femoral, carotid, brachial pulses) gives a subjective indication of SV; as SV decreases, so does the pulse amplitude. In progressive circulatory failure, the pulse amplitude diminishes, becomes weak and thready before finally, it is impalpable. Simultaneous palpation and comparison of central and peripheral pulses (e.g. radial and carotid) may be useful. Peripheral pulses decrease in amplitude earlier than central ones. Note that caution is required in their interpretation when vasoconstriction is present (e.g. ambient temperature is low, or in an anxious or pyrexial child).

The presence or absence of peripheral pulses is neither a specific nor sensitive indicator of circulatory compromise, but is useful in conjunction with other clinical signs. However, **diminishing central pulses are a pre-terminal sign**, indicating that cardiorespiratory arrest is imminent.

Capillary refill and skin colour

The skin of a healthy child is warm to touch unless the ambient temperature is low. Their capillary refill time (CRT) is normally < 2 seconds, but when there is decreased skin perfusion, the CRT is prolonged.

Evaluation of CRT is best performed by applying cutaneous pressure on the centre of the sternum for 5 seconds. Following removal of the pressure, the blanching of the skin should disappear within 2 seconds. A slower refill time (i.e. prolonged CRT) is indicative of poor skin perfusion. A pyrexial child with hypovolaemia will have a prolonged CRT, despite having a raised body temperature. A low ambient temperature or poor local lighting conditions reduces the accuracy of CRT. The CRT should be considered in context of the accompanying cardiovascular signs.

Initially, hypoxia produces vasoconstriction and hence the child appears pale. As their clinical condition deteriorates, the child's colour becomes mottled and ultimately cyanosed. Cyanosis due to circulatory failure is initially peripheral, whereas hypoxaemia due to respiratory failure results in central cyanosis.

Peripheral vasoconstriction and decreased perfusion may also be indicated by a demarcation line between warm and cold skin. This can be detected by running the back of your hand up the child's limb. The demarcation line will travel towards the trunk over time if the child's condition is deteriorating, and vice versa if it is improving.

Blood pressure

In most forms of shock, the BP is initially maintained within the normal range (Table 2.5) for the child as a result of the body's compensatory mechanisms (e.g. tachycardia, vasoconstriction, increased myocardial contractility). Only when compensation is no longer possible, does hypotension occur and a decompensated state results.

Table 2.5 Normal and lower limit of systolic blood pressure by age

Age	Systolic blood pressure (mmHg)	
	Normal	Lower limit
0 – 1 month	> 60	50 – 60
1 – 12 months	80	70
1 – 10 years	90 + (2 x age in years)	70 + (2 x age in years)
> 10 years	120	90

In hypovolaemia, approximately 40% of the child's total circulating volume can be lost before hypotension occurs. This means that BP only drops at a late stage in hypovolaemia (e.g. trauma, diarrhoeal illness, gut necrosis). It is therefore important that compensated circulatory failure is detected and managed at an early stage, i.e. before BP drops and decompensation occurs.

In children over 1 year, BP limits can be estimated by the formulae in Table 2.5.

In neonates, the lower limit for systolic BP is 50-60 mmHg and for infants, from 1-12 months, it is 70 mmHg.

Regardless of the method used to obtain the BP (auscultatory or oscillometric) it is important that the appropriate cuff size is used. The cuff width should be > 80% of the child's upper arm length, and the bladder cover more than 40% of the circumference of their arm. The same size cuff should be used on each occasion that the BP is measured.

Hypotension is a sign of physiological decompensation and indicates imminent cardiorespiratory arrest.

Effects of circulatory inadequacy on other body organs

Ongoing circulatory compromise rapidly affects other body organs/systems:

Respiratory system

The metabolic acidosis that results from circulatory compromise leads to tachypnoea. However, there will not initially be other signs of increased work of breathing.

Conscious level

Hypoxia and/or hypercapnia initially lead to agitation and/or drowsiness. Progressive cerebral hypoxia ultimately results in loss of consciousness. In infants and young children, initial cerebral hypoxia may be difficult to detect but their parents/carers frequently report that the baby/child is not responding to them as usual and, as in respiratory failure, this information should not be ignored. The level of consciousness should be assessed by the AVPU score.

Generalised hypotonia also accompanies cerebral hypoxia.

Urine output

Information regarding the degree of reduced renal perfusion can be obtained by measuring the output of urine. A urinary output of < 2 ml kg^{-1} h^{-1} in infants or < 1 ml kg^{-1} h^{-1} in children older than 1 year, is an indication of inadequate renal perfusion. Asking parents/carers about the child's urine output (e.g. the number of wet nappies) may reveal a history of oliguria or anuria.

Management of circulatory compromise

The treatment of circulatory problems is dependent on achieving a patent airway and effectively managing ventilation with appropriate delivery of high-flow oxygen before turning attention to circulatory procedures.

Immediately life-threatening causes of circulatory failure (e.g. massive or continuing haemorrhage, tension pneumothorax) must be sought and urgently treated.

Insertion of at least one large bore vascular cannula should be performed rapidly. This can be achieved by either intravenous or intraosseous routes.

Unless contraindicated (e.g. cardiac failure) volume replacement should be started using 20 ml kg^{-1} boluses of isotonic salt solution, i.e. 0.9% saline. Glucose containing fluids with low sodium levels should NEVER be used for resuscitation, only to correct for low blood glucose levels.

The use of vasoactive medications may be needed (circulatory access procedures, fluids and medications are looked at in Chapter 6).

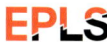

Signs of cardiorespiratory failure include alteration of consciousness, hypotonia, tachycardia, decreased central pulses and absent peripheral pulses. Bradycardia, hypotension, bradypnoea, gasping and apnoea are terminal events preceding imminent cardiorespiratory arrest.

If any of the following signs are present, immediate intervention should be undertaken:

- Coma or alteration of consciousness
- Exhaustion
- Cyanosis
- Tachypnoea (RR > 60 min^{-1})
- HR < 100 min^{-1} for newborn
- HR > 180 min^{-1} or < 80 min^{-1} before 1 year
- HR > 160 min^{-1} or < 60 min^{-1} after 1 year
- Seizures

A rapid assessment must be made of every child in whom respiratory, circulatory or cardiorespiratory failure is suspected.

D: Disability – Central neurological assessment

Following the appropriate management of the child's airway, ventilation and circulation, their neurological status should be evaluated.

Whilst both respiratory and circulatory failure can have central neurological effects, some neurological conditions (e.g. status epilepticus, meningitis or raised intracranial pressure) may affect the respiratory and circulatory systems.

Neurological function

Conscious level

A rapid assessment of the child's conscious level can be determined by the AVPU score.

If required, the painful stimulus should be delivered either by applying pressure to the supraorbital ridge or rubbing the sternum. A child who is unresponsive to painful (P) stimuli has a significant degree of neurological derangement equivalent to a Glasgow coma scale score of 8 or less.

Pupils

The size and reactivity of pupils can be affected by a number of things, including medications and cerebral lesions. Important signs to look for are dilatation, inequality and non-reactivity of the child's pupils. These features potentially indicate serious brain dysfunction.

Posture

Seriously ill children become hypotonic and floppy. However, if there is serious brain dysfunction, stiff posturing may be demonstrated. This posturing (which may only be evident when a painful stimulus is applied) can be decorticate (flexed arms and extended legs) or decerebrate (extended arms and legs); both indicate serious brain dysfunction.

Respiratory effects of central neurological failure

Comatose children with brain dysfunction may exhibit abnormal respiratory patterns e.g. hyperventilation, Cheyne-Stoke respiratory pattern (alternate periods of hyperventilation and apnoea) or complete apnoea.

Circulatory effects of central neurological failure

Raised intracranial pressure causes the Cushing's triad (abnormal breathing pattern with bradycardia and hypertension). **This is a late and pre-terminal sign of neurological failure.**

E: Exposure

To ensure that no additional significant clinical information (e.g. rashes) is missed, it is vital to examine the child fully by exposing their body. Appropriate measures to minimise heat loss (especially in infants) and respect dignity must be adopted at all times.

The ABCDE approach

In all seriously ill or injured children, the underlying principles of assessment, initial management and ongoing reassessments are the same. They are based on the systematic ABCDE approach (Table 2.6):

A	**Airway**
B	**Breathing**
C	**Circulation**
D	**Disability (mental status)**
E	**Exposure**

General principles of the ABCDE approach

- Ensure personal safety
- Observe the child generally to determine the overall level of illness (i.e. do they look seriously unwell; are they interacting with parents/care givers)
- Speak to the child and assess the appropriateness of their response; ask the parents about the child's 'usual' behaviour
- If they are unconscious and unresponsive to your voice, administer tactile stimulation. If they respond by speaking or crying, this indicates that they have a patent airway,

Table 2.6 Specific assessments and actions in initial ABCDE approach

Assessment	Information sought	Possible resultant actions
On approaching the child	Note: • General appearance • Interaction with parent/caregiver	
A Airway patency	Is the airway: • Patent (i.e. conscious, vocalising) • At risk • Obstructed	• Suction if indicated • Head positioning • Oropharyngeal airway • Reassess • Summon expert help
B Breathing adequacy	Note/observe/perform: • Conscious level • Air movement (look, listen, feel) • Respiratory rate • Chest expansion • Use of accessory muscles/recessions • Palpation • Percussion • Auscultation • SpO_2 and FiO_2	• Administer high-flow oxygen appropriately • Support breathing with bag-mask ventilation (BMV) as necessary • Reassess • Summon expert help
C Circulation adequacy	Note/observe/perform: • Evidence of haemorrhage/fluid loss • Conscious level • Heart rate • Capillary refill time • Presence of distal/central pulses • Pulse volume features • Skin temperature and colour • Blood pressure • Urine output	• Control any external bleeding • Attach monitoring (as appropriate to setting) • Obtain circulatory access (IV or IO) • Estimate weight • Blood samples for laboratory testing and bedside glucose estimation • Fluid bolus (20 ml kg^{-1}) • Reassess • Summon expert help
D Disability (conscious level)	Note: • AVPU score • Interaction with parent and surroundings • Posture and muscle tone • Pupil size and reactivity	• Reconsider A, B and C management as conscious level dictates • Establish bedside glucose estimation • Establish if any medications have been given/possibly ingested • Reassess • Summon expert help
E Exposure	Note/observe: • Evidence of any blood loss/skin lesions/wounds/drains/rashes etc • Core temperature	• Reconsider specific management e.g. antibiotics in sepsis • Consider appropriate temperature control measures • Reassess • Summon expert help

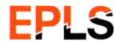

are breathing and have cerebral perfusion. Regardless of the child's response to initial stimulation, you should move on to full assessment of ABCDE

- Appropriate high-flow oxygen delivery should be commenced immediately

- Vital sign monitoring should be requested early (ECG, SpO_2 and non-invasive BP monitoring)

- Circulatory access should be achieved as soon as possible. Blood test investigations and a bedside glucose estimation should be obtained

> **Key learning points**
>
> ▸ Early recognition of the seriously ill child prevents the majority of cardiorespiratory arrests, thus reducing morbidity and mortality
>
> ▸ The structured ABCDE approach helps ensure that potentially life-threatening problems are identified and dealt with in order of priority

Further reading

Brierley J, Carcillo JA, Choong K, Cornell T et al. Clinical practice parameters for hemodynamic support of pediatric and neonatal septic shock: 2007 update from the American College of Critical Care Medicine. Critical Care Medicine 2009; 37(2):666-688.

Carcillo JA. Pediatric septic shock and multiple organ failure. Crit Care Clin 2003; 19:413-40.

De Man SA, Andre JL, Bachmann H et al. Blood pressure in childhood: pooled findings of six European studies. J Hypertension. 1991; 9:109-114.

de Oliveira CF, de Oliveira DS, Gottschald AF, et al. ACCM/PALS haemodynamic support guidelines for paediatric septic shock: an outcomes comparison with and without monitoring central venous oxygen saturation. Intensive Care Med 2008;34:1065–75.

Lafey JG, Kavanagh BP. Hypocapnia. N Engl J Med. 2002; 347:43-53.

Levin DL, Morriss F. Essentials of Pediatric Intensive Care. Quality Medical Publishing, St. Louis, USA, 1990.

Plum F, Posner JB. The diagnostic of stupor and coma, 3rd edition. FA Davis Co, Philadelphia, USA, 1982.

Pollack MM, Fields AI, Rutimann UE et al. Sequential cardiopulmonary variables in pediatric survivors and nonsurvivors of septic shock. Crit Care Med. 1984; 12:554-559.

Basic Life Support

CHAPTER 3

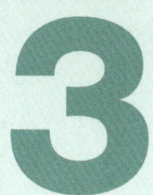

Learning outcomes

To understand:

- ▶ The importance of early effective basic life support (BLS) for decreasing mortality and morbidity
- ▶ How and when to activate the Emergency Medical Service (EMS) or the in-hospital clinical emergency team
- ▶ The rationale for the sequence of steps in BLS
- ▶ The importance of early appropriate choking management
- ▶ The rationale for the different techniques of BLS employed in infants and children

Age definitions

For the purposes of basic life support (BLS), an infant is a baby < 1 year and a child is aged between 1 year and puberty. It is neither appropriate nor necessary to formally establish the onset of puberty; if the rescuer thinks the victim is a child, they should use the paediatric guidelines.

Introduction

BLS is the combination of manoeuvres and skills that, without the use of technical adjuncts, provides recognition and management of a person in cardiac or respiratory arrest and 'buys time' until the victim can receive more advanced treatment.

BLS must be started as rapidly as possible. Its main objective is to achieve sufficient oxygenation to 'protect' the brain and other vital organs. Ideally, all citizens should possess BLS knowledge and skills. The sequence of actions in BLS is known as cardiopulmonary resuscitation (CPR). BLS is more effective when the rescuer is proficient in its delivery, but even suboptimal CPR gives a better result than no CPR at all. Hence rescuers unable or unwilling to provide mouth-to-mouth ventilation should be encouraged to perform at least compression-only CPR.

BLS can be executed without any adjuncts but expired air ventilation provides only 16-17% of oxygen. Oxygen should be given as soon as possible. The trained healthcare provider must provide bag-mask ventilation with oxygen as soon as the necessary equipment is available.

Background

In the management of the collapsed child, a number of factors are critical in maximising the chances of a good outcome. The most important is the early recognition and appropriate intervention in children who exhibit signs of respiratory and/or circulatory compromise. Prevention of cardiorespiratory arrest by the optimal management of respiratory distress and/or circulatory failure will improve the prognosis (Chapter 1).

Nevertheless, there will always be some children in whom respiratory and/or circulatory collapse cannot be prevented. For these children, early BLS, rapid activation of the Emergency Medical Service (EMS) or in-hospital clinical emergency team, and prompt, effective advanced life support are crucial in improving mortality and morbidity.

BLS sequence

The single lay rescuer should follow the adult sequence for children except that they should (ideally) deliver 5 initial rescue breaths and perform 1 minute of CPR before going for help.

The BLS algorithm (Figure 3.1) and sequence described below is for **healthcare providers** who may occasionally start BLS alone but would normally work in a team.

Although unusual, primary cardiac arrest in ventricular fibrillation or pulseless ventricular tachycardia does occasionally occur in children. If this situation is likely, such as with the sudden, witnessed collapse of a child with a known cardiac condition, optimal outcome will depend on early defibrillation. It is then preferable for a lone rescuer to activate the EMS before starting BLS and to use an AED, if available.

However, for the majority of children who suffer cardiorespiratory arrest, the recommended sequence of events is based on two facts:

1. Cardiorespiratory arrest is hypoxic in origin and therefore the priority is prompt oxygenation (provided by rescue breaths)

2. The most common cardiac arrhythmia is profound bradycardia deteriorating into asystole; hence effective BLS is more important than access to a defibrillator

It is important that rescuers follow the specific order of steps in BLS because if one manoeuvre is missed or incorrectly performed, the effectiveness of the next step is likely to also be compromised (Figure 3.2).

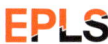

Chapter 3 Basic Life Support

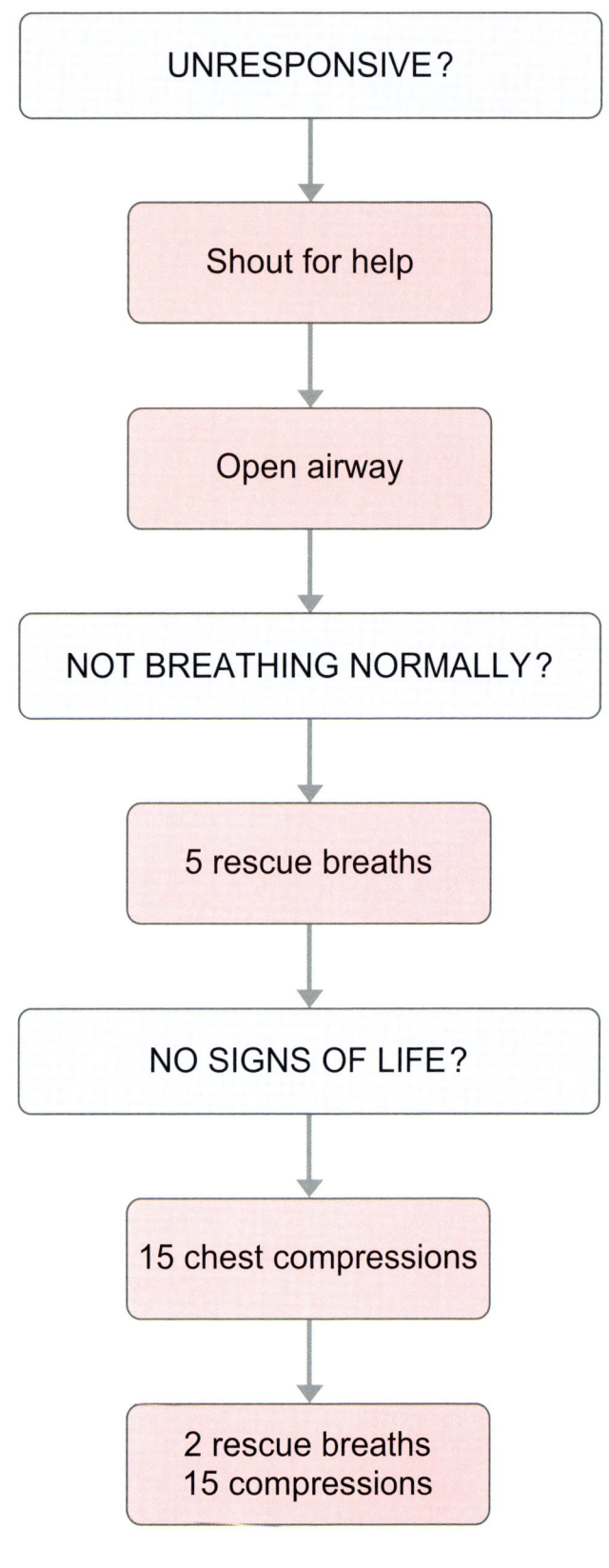

Figure 3.1 Paediatric BLS algorithm

- S Safety
- S Stimulate
- S Shout for assistance
- A Airway
- B Breathing
- C Circulation
- R Reassess

Figure 3.2 BLS sequence

S – Safety

In all emergencies it is essential to quickly assess the situation and ensure the safety of first the rescuer(s) and then that of the child; although the potential hazards may be different, this is equally important whether the situation occurs within or outside the healthcare environment.

All bodily fluids should be treated as potentially infectious; put on gloves as soon as practicable and use barrier devices for ventilation (e.g. pocket mask) if possible. Whilst the efficacy of face shields is uncertain and they may not reliably prevent transmission of infection, their use affords some protection and may make it more acceptable for the receipt or delivery of rescue breaths.

On approaching the child, and before touching them, rapidly look for any clues as to what may have caused the emergency as this may influence the way the child is managed (e.g. any suspicion of head or neck injury necessitates consideration of cervical spine immobilisation).

S – Stimulate

It is important to establish the responsiveness of the apparently unconscious child by tactile and verbal stimulation as they may not be in a critical condition. You can do this by stabilising the child's head by placing one hand on their forehead and then tugging their hair, whilst calling their name or telling them to "wake up". Never shake a child vigorously.

If the child responds (e.g. moves, cries or talks), his clinical status and any further potential dangers should be assessed, and if necessary, help obtained.

If there is no response continue with BLS as described below.

S – Shout

If there is only one rescuer, they must not leave the child (or delay BLS to use a mobile telephone), but shout "help" as they start BLS. If there is another person present, they should be asked to summon the EMS.

This second rescuer should get help by dialling 999 or 112 for the EMS if out of hospital, or 2222 for the hospital clinical emergency team. They must be able to convey the specific information listed in Table 3.1.

Table 3.1 Information required when requesting EMS	
National 999 or 112 ambulance request	In-hospital 2222 request
Precise location of the emergency	Precise location of the emergency
Type of emergency (e.g. infant in cardiorespiratory arrest, child in road traffic accident)	Specific clinical emergency team required (e.g. paediatric, paediatric trauma)
Number and age of victim(s)	Any other local policy requirements
Severity and urgency of the situation	

The caller should only end the phone call once the operator confirms no further information is needed. They should then return to the rescuer(s) delivering BLS and inform them that the EMS has been activated. If the event is within a healthcare environment, appropriate clinical emergency equipment should also be taken to the patient.

A – Airway

In the unconscious child, the tongue is likely to at least partly occlude their airway. This can usually be overcome by using a head tilt and chin lift manoeuvre or, if necessary, by performing a jaw thrust.

Head tilt and chin lift

This is a simple and effective initial manoeuvre. To perform the head tilt, approach the child from the side, place one hand on their forehead and gently tilt their head back. In infants, the head should be placed in a neutral position (Figure 3.3). For the child, a 'sniffing' position that causes some extension of the head on the neck will be required (Figure 3.4).

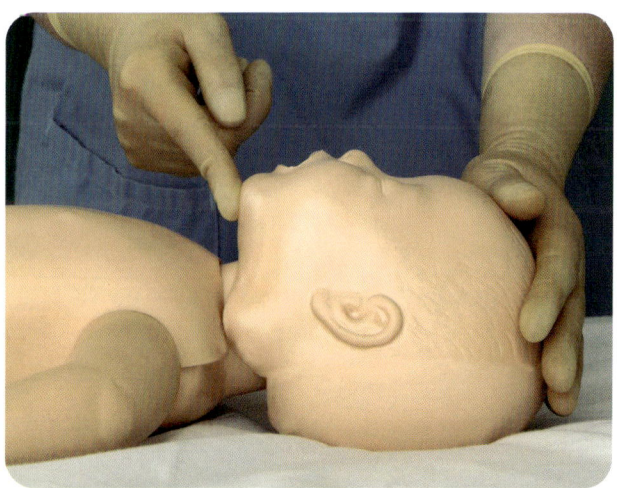

Figure 3.3 Head tilt and chin lift in an infant (neutral head position)

EUROPEAN PAEDIATRIC LIFE SUPPORT

Chapter 3 Basic Life Support

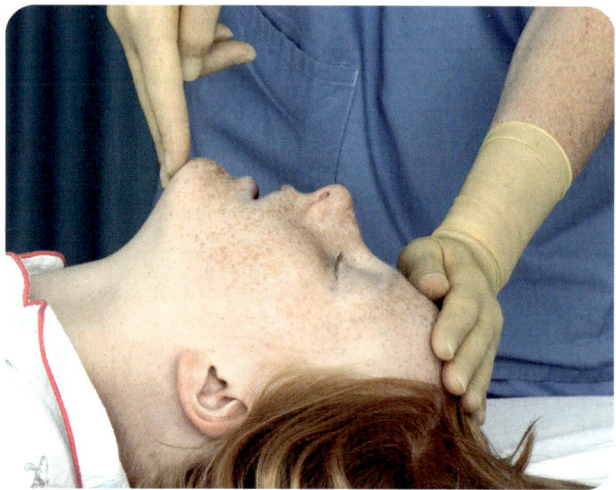

Figure 3.4 Head tilt and chin lift in a child ('sniffing' position)

The chin lift is performed by placing the fingertips of the rescuer's other hand on the bony part of the child's lower jaw, and lifting the chin upwards. It is essential that the rescuer takes care not to compress the soft tissues under the child's jaw as this will occlude the airway.

Jaw thrust

This is the most effective airway opening manoeuvre in children and the preferred method when cervical spine immobilisation is required. To perform a jaw thrust, the rescuer should approach the child from behind, and place their hands on either side of the child's head. Two or three fingertips of both hands should be placed under both angles of the child's lower jaw. With their thumbs resting gently on the child's cheeks, the rescuer should then lift the jaw upwards. The rescuers elbows should rest on the surface that the child is laid on (Figure 3.5).

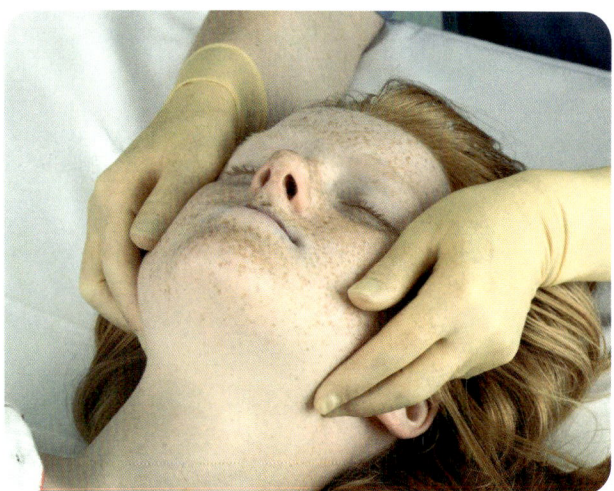

Figure 3.5 Jaw thrust manoeuvre in a child

Whichever method of airway opening is used, it is also important for rescuers to look in the child's mouth to ensure there is no obvious foreign body present. If a foreign body is seen and the rescuer is confident that they can remove it with a single finger sweep, this can be attempted. However, blind finger sweeps should never be performed. The management of choking is discussed later in this chapter.

B – Breathing

Assessing for normal breathing

After opening the airway, the rescuer needs to assess the child for effective, normal breathing. The best way to do this is to 'look, listen and feel' whilst maintaining the airway opening manoeuvre.

LOOK	for chest (and abdominal) movements
LISTEN	for airflow at the mouth and nose (+/- additional noises)
FEEL	for airflow at the mouth and nose

The rescuer positions themselves with a cheek just a few centimetres above the child's mouth and nose, and looks along the child's body for **no more than 10 seconds** (Figures 3.6 and 3.7).

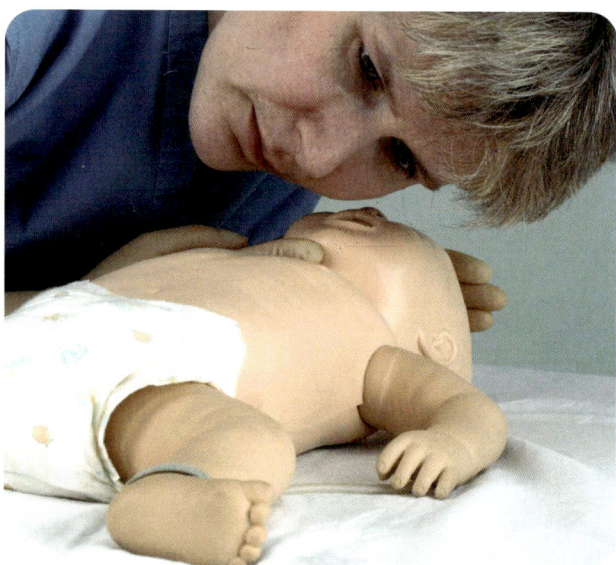

Figure 3.6 Checking for breathing in an infant

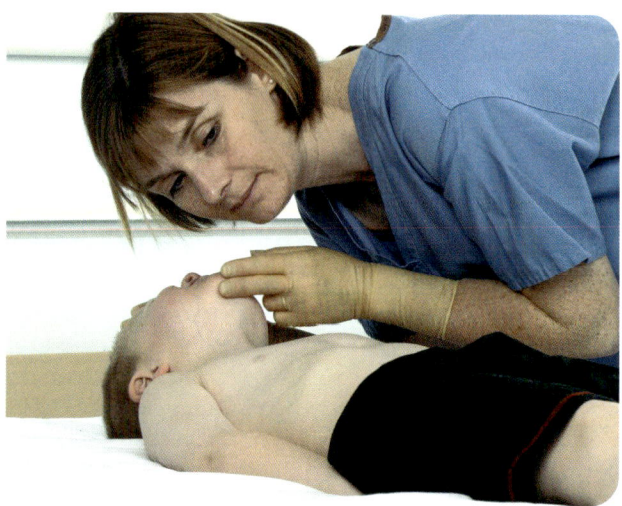

Figure 3.7 Checking for breathing in a child

If the child is breathing normally and effectively, the rescuer should maintain the airway opening manoeuvre whilst help is summoned. However, if there is no-one else to activate the EMS, the rescuer must do this themselves. Unless contraindicated (i.e. suspicion of spinal injury) the child should be placed in the recovery position (described later in this chapter) until further help arrives.

If the child is not breathing normally, or they are only gasping ineffectively (agonal breathing), the rescuer must immediately give rescue breaths. Agonal breathing is infrequent or irregular, noisy gasps, which must not be confused with normal breathing.

Delivery of expired air rescue breaths

The aim of rescue breaths is to deliver oxygen to the child's lungs. Until an appropriate ventilation device is available, expired air rescue breathing is required. This will provide approximately 16-17% oxygen. The effectiveness of rescue breaths is assessed by observing the rise and fall of the child's chest wall; rescuers may need to adapt the pressure and volume of breath delivery to the individual child to ensure that chest movement is obtained with each breath delivered.

Five initial rescue breaths should be given. Each breath should be delivered slowly (over approximately 1-1.5 seconds). This maximises the amount of oxygen delivered to the child's lungs and minimises the risk of gastric distension. By inhaling deeply themselves between giving each rescue breath, the rescuer can optimise the oxygen and minimise the carbon dioxide levels they deliver to the child. The effectiveness of the rescue breaths can only be determined by observing the rise and fall of the chest. The rescuer must adapt the pressure and volume of exhalation to the characteristics of the child to ensure that chest movement is seen with each breath given.

If chest movement is not observed with attempted delivery of a rescue breath, the rescuer must reassess the child's airway (i.e. reposition the child's head) and ensure they have an adequate seal between their mouth and the child's face before they attempt the next breath. If, despite repositioning the child's head and having an adequate seal, the rescuer is still unable to achieve movement of the child's chest, the likelihood of choking should be considered and the rescuer should move straight to chest compressions.

Mouth-to-mouth and nose rescue breathing

This is the recommended technique for giving expired air rescue breaths to an infant. The rescuer places their mouth around both the mouth and nose to create a tight seal, and then blows into the infant (Figure 3.8). If it is not possible to cover both the mouth and nose, the rescuer can choose to blow into either the infant's mouth or nose (with the nostrils occluded or the mouth closed, to minimise escape of air).

Mouth-to-mouth rescue breathing

This is the recommended technique for giving expired air rescue breaths to a child (Figure 3.9). The rescuer places their mouth over the child's mouth, creating a seal. Using the fingers of their hand at the top of the child's head, the

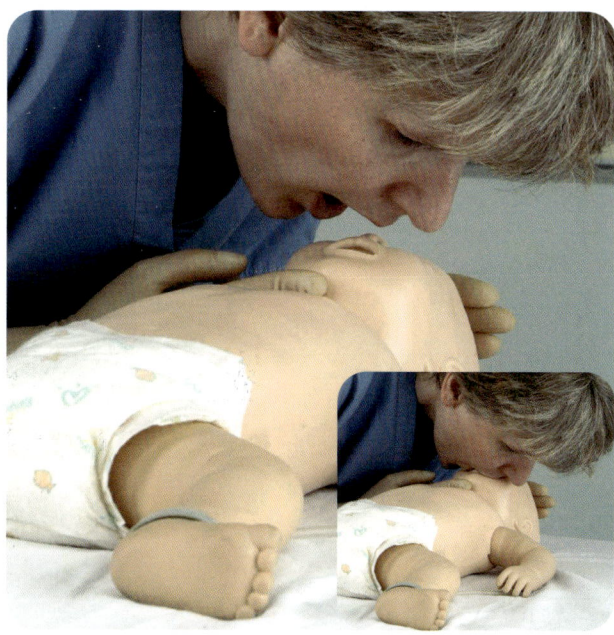

Figure 3.8 Mouth-to-mouth and nose rescue breath delivery in an infant

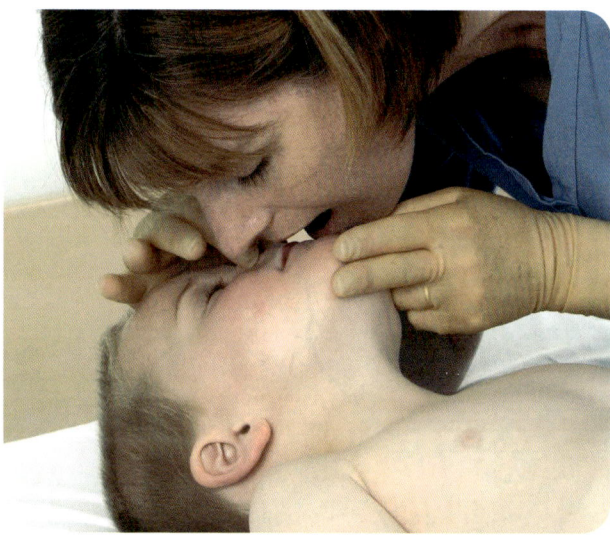

Figure 3.9 Mouth-to-mouth rescue breath delivery in a child

rescuer occludes the child's nostrils to ensure that the rescue breath does not escape through the child's nose.

C – Circulation

Assessing for 'signs of life'

After the 5 initial rescue breaths attempts are given, the rescuer needs to determine whether the child has an adequate spontaneous circulation, or if they also require chest compressions. The time taken for any rescuer to assess the circulation should **not exceed 10 seconds**.

Observe the child for 'signs of life' (i.e. swallowing, vocalising, coughing or normal [not agonal] breathing).

For healthcare professionals who are trained in pulse checking, a central pulse can be palpated, whilst simultaneously looking for 'signs of life'.

Chapter 3 Basic Life Support

In infants the recommended sites for central pulse palpation are the femoral or brachial artery (Figure 3.10). In the child it is the femoral or carotid artery (Figure 3.11).

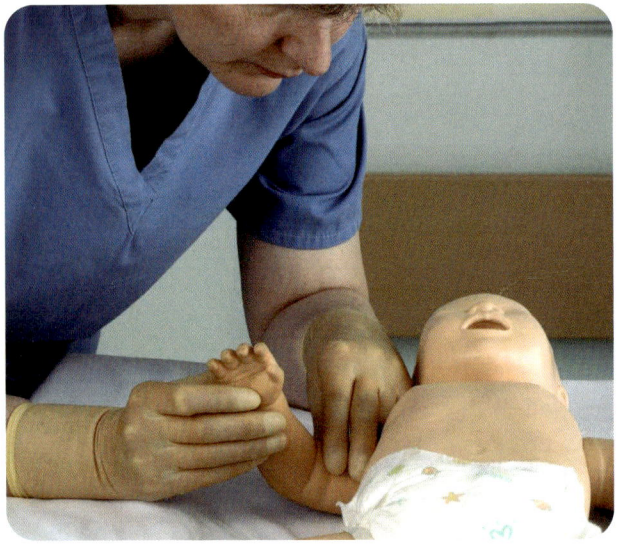

Figure 3.10 Brachial pulse palpation on an infant

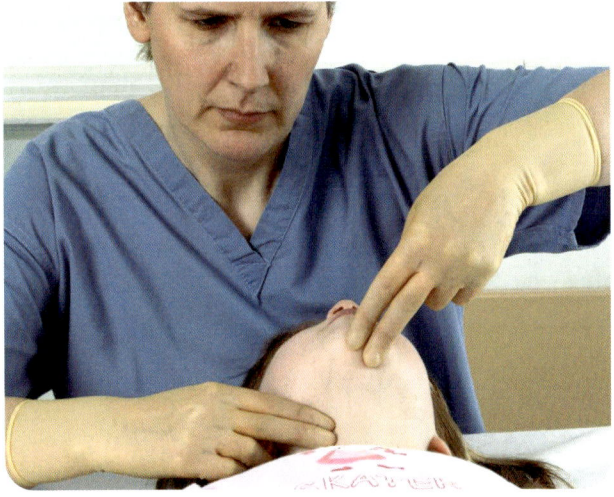

Figure 3.11 Carotid pulse palpation on a child

If there are no 'signs of life', chest compressions should be started immediately, unless the rescuer is **CERTAIN** they can feel a definite pulse > 60 min^{-1} **within 10 seconds**. If there is any doubt, start chest compressions.

If there are 'signs of life' and/or a pulse is found (i.e. > 60 min^{-1}), the rescuer should reassess the child's breathing. If breathing is absent or inadequate (e.g. agonal breathing) then rescue breathing should be continued at a rate of 12-20 breaths min^{-1}. The child's breathing and circulation should be frequently reassessed and BLS continued until either the EMS arrives to take over, or until the child starts to breathe spontaneously.

If effective spontaneous breathing is established, and there is no suspicion of cervical spine trauma, the child should be placed in a safe, side-lying position (page 27).

Principles of chest compressions

Chest compressions are serial, rhythmic compressions of the anterior chest wall, intended to cause blood to flow to vital organ tissues in an attempt to keep them viable until return of spontaneous circulation (ROSC) is achieved.

The recommended ratio of chest compressions to ventilations for infants and children is 15:2. However, a lone healthcare professional may choose to use the standard adult ratio of 30:2 to avoid changing frequently between rescue breathing and chest compression. For simplicity, lay persons are taught to use the adult 30:2 ratio. Whichever ratio is used, chest compressions must be performed effectively.

The rate of chest compressions should be 100-120 min^{-1}; it should be noted that when interspersed with rescue breaths, the actual number of compressions delivered will be less than this.

Effective chest compression is facilitated by ensuring the child is lying on a firm flat surface. It also requires depression of the child's chest by at least one third of the anteroposterior diameter, with approximately equal time spent in the compression and relaxation phases.

During the relaxation phase of each compression, the rescuer should release the pressure whilst leaving their hand(s)/fingers in position on the child's chest wall.

At the end of each series of chest compressions, the hand(s)/fingers must be removed from the child's chest in order to effectively perform airway opening manoeuvres and give two rescue breaths.

Landmarking for chest compressions

In all infants and children, deliver chest compressions over the lower half of the sternum. In order to avoid compressing the upper abdomen, locate the xiphisternum at the angle where the lower costal margins meet and compress one finger's breadth above this point (Figure 3.12 and Figure 3.13).

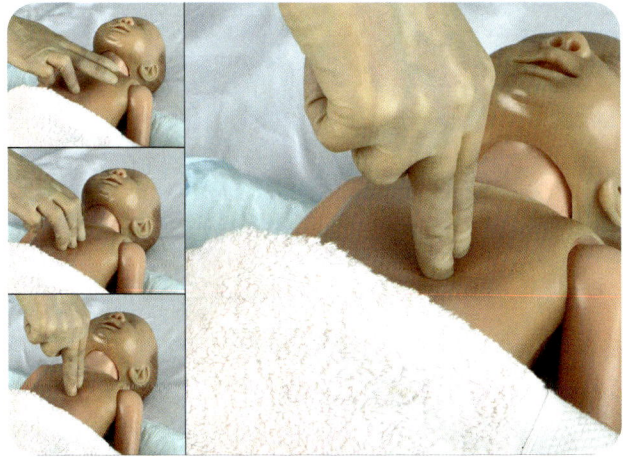

Figure 3.12 Landmarking for chest compressions on an infant

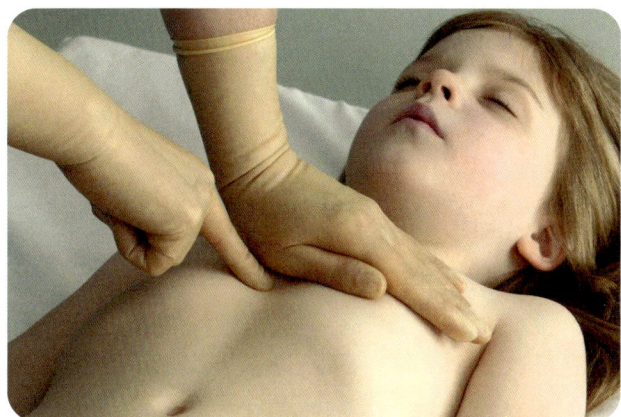

Figure 3.13 Landmarking for chest compressions on a child

Performing chest compressions

Infant chest compression

Two-finger technique

This is the recommended method of infant chest compression for the lone rescuer. Having landmarked as described above, place two fingers of one hand in the correct position on the sternum and depress it by at least one third of the anteroposterior diameter (Figure 3.14 and Figure 3.15).

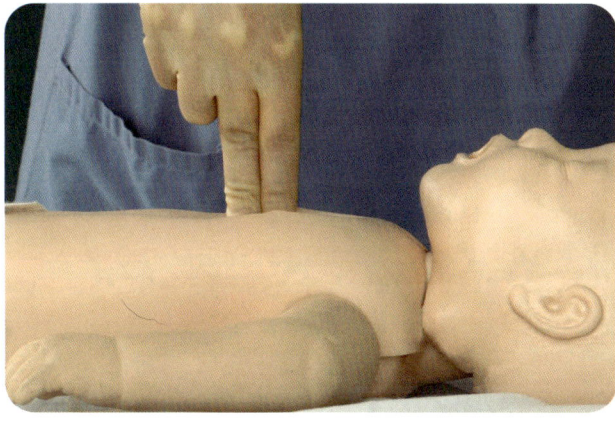

Figure 3.14 Two-finger chest compression on an infant – depression phase

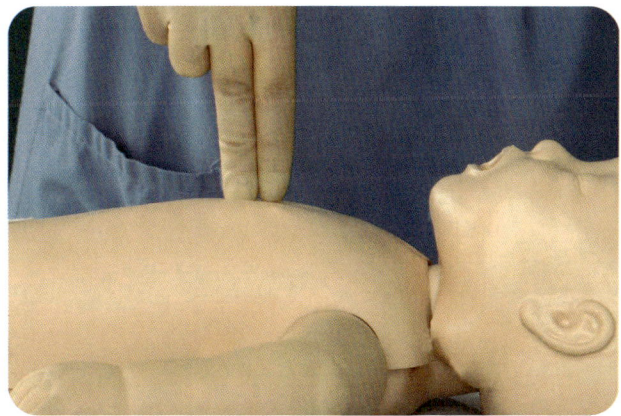

Figure 3.15 Two-finger chest compression on an infant – relaxation phase

Two-thumb encircling technique

This is the recommended method of infant chest compression for two rescuers. There is evidence that this method delivers greater cardiac output than the two-finger technique, but it is difficult for a single rescuer to perform and also deliver rescue breaths in a timely and effective manner. It is therefore usually reserved for in-hospital resuscitation where there are two rescuers and ventilation delivery devices can be used.

The two-thumb encircling technique requires a healthcare professional to be positioned at the infant's head to maintain the airway and deliver ventilation. A second rescuer, at the infant's side (or at their feet), places their two thumbs side-by-side in the correct position on the lower half of the sternum (Figure 3.16). In a very small baby, the thumbs may be placed one on top of the other. The rest of the rescuer's hands are then able to support the infant's back as they encircle the chest wall. Chest compressions are delivered as described previously.

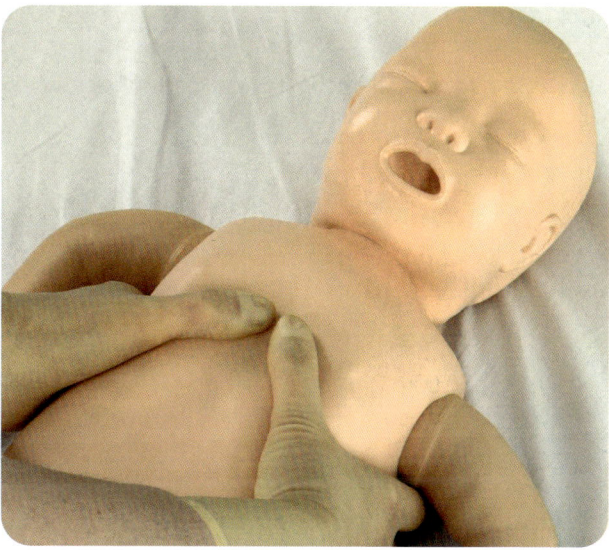

Figure 3.16 Two-thumb encircling chest compressions on an infant

Child chest compression

Having landmarked as previously described, the rescuer should position themselves at one side of the child, and place the heel of one hand along the long axis of the lower half of the child's sternum. The fingers should be raised off the chest so that pressure is exerted only through the heel of the hand and on to the sternum.

By positioning themselves so that their elbow is locked straight, and their shoulders are directly over the heel of their hand on the child's chest, the rescuer can use their body weight to depress the sternum to the required depth. If it is difficult to achieve a depth of at least one third of the child's anteroposterior chest diameter, the rescuer should use both hands; the second one placed on top of the first, with the fingers linked together off the chest wall (Figure 3.17).

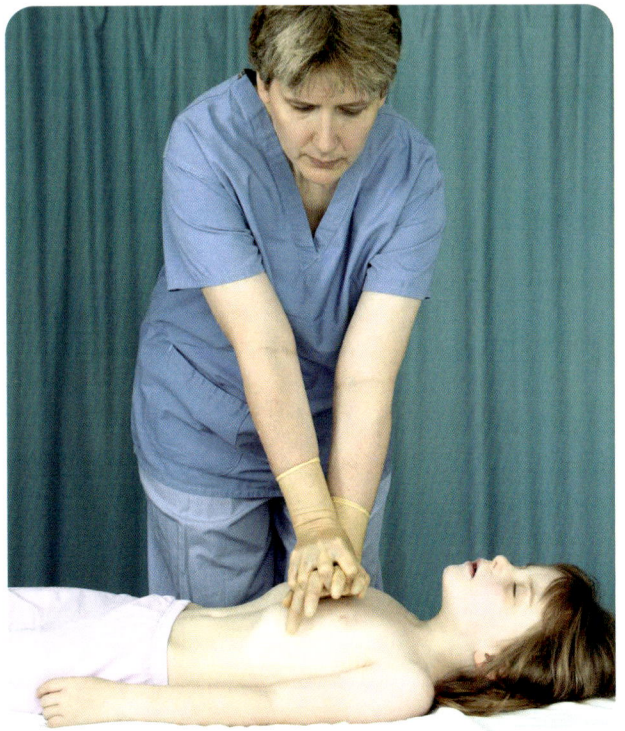

Figure 3.17 Two-handed chest compression on a child

R – Reassess

After approximately one minute of BLS, a single rescuer should briefly stop to establish whether or not someone has called the EMS. If this has not occurred (or they are uncertain) the single rescuer must now call for more help.

Use a mobile phone if available. Otherwise, if the victim is an infant or a very small child, the rescuer may be able to carry him safely to activate a telephone to summon further assistance, and then continue CPR. If the means of summoning help is some distance away, the rescuer should try to provide CPR while going to the phone. If the child is too large to carry, leave the child to activate the EMS, and return to recommence BLS as soon as possible.

If the EMS has already been activated, the rescuer should immediately resume BLS unless there are obvious 'signs of life'.

Continuation of BLS

BLS should only be stopped when:

- the child exhibits adequate 'signs of life'
- further rescuers take over resuscitation
- the single rescuer is too exhausted to continue

As soon as the EMS and/or appropriate paediatric resuscitation equipment becomes available, advanced life support techniques can start.

Choking

When a foreign body enters their airway, a child will react immediately by coughing in an attempt to expel it. A child who is choking on a foreign body but is still able to cough effectively must be actively encouraged to do so. A spontaneous cough is not only safer, but it is probably more effective than any manoeuvre a rescuer might perform.

However, if coughing is absent or becoming ineffective, the child's airway is at risk of complete obstruction, which will rapidly result in asphyxiation. Any child who is unable to effectively cough as a result of foreign body aspiration, requires immediate interventions (Figure 3.18).

Recognition of choking

Choking is characterised by the sudden onset of respiratory distress associated with coughing, gagging or stridor.

The majority of choking events in infants and children occur during play or feeding, and are therefore frequently witnessed by an adult which means interventions can start immediately. However, it is important to be aware that the signs and symptoms of choking (Table 3.2) can be confused with those of other causes of airway obstruction (e.g. laryngitis or epiglottitis) which require different management.

Table 3.2 Signs of choking

General signs

Witnessed episode

Coughing or choking

Sudden onset

Recent history of playing with, or eating small objects

Ineffective cough	Effective cough
Unable to vocalise	Crying or verbal response to questions
Quiet or silent cough	Loud cough
Unable to breathe	Able to take a breath before coughing
Cyanosis	Fully responsive
Decreasing level of consciousness	

Management of choking

As with BLS, it is essential to quickly assess the situation and ensure the safety of first the rescuer(s) and then that of the child; although the potential hazards are different, this is equally important whether the situation occurs within or outside of the healthcare environment.

If the child is coughing effectively, no external manoeuvre is necessary. The rescuer should encourage the child's coughing and observe them closely.

If the child's coughing is absent or becoming ineffective, the rescuer must shout for help and quickly determine the child's conscious level.

Conscious infants and children

If the child is conscious but their coughing is absent or ineffective, the rescuer must give back blows. These are intended to loosen the object for the child to be able to then

Paediatric Choking Treatment Algorithm

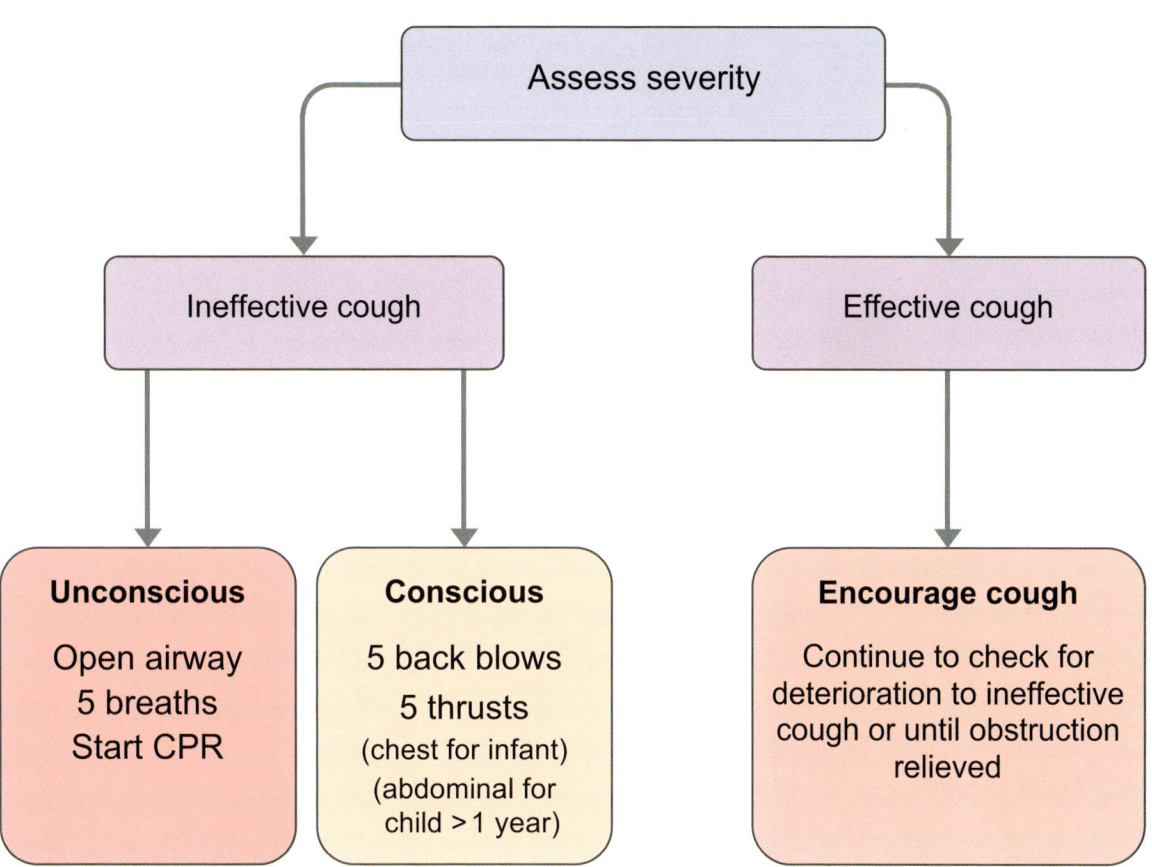

Figure 3.18 Management of Choking

expel it. If back blows do not relieve the airway obstruction, *thrusts* should be given; chest thrusts for infants and abdominal thrusts for children. These thrusts are intended as an 'artificial cough'; they increase the intrathoracic pressure which will facilitate expulsion of the foreign body.

Delivery of back blows to an infant

1. To give back blows safely, the rescuer should either sit on a chair or kneel on the floor, and hold the infant in a head downwards, prone position across their lap (Figure 3.19).

2. The rescuer must support the infant's head by placing the thumb of one hand at the angle of the lower jaw, and one or two fingers from the same hand at the same point on the other side of the infant's face. Care must be taken not to compress the soft tissues under the infant's jaw.

3. Up to 5 sharp blows should be delivered to the middle of the infant's back, between their scapulae, with the heel of the rescuer's other hand.

The aim is to relieve the obstruction with each individual back blow rather than to give all 5.

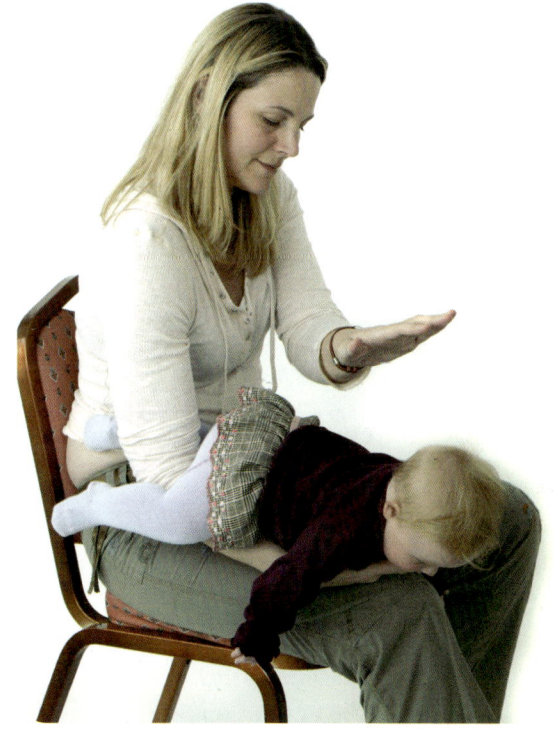

Figure 3.19 Delivery of back blows to an infant

Delivery of back blows to a child

1. To maximise effectiveness, the rescuer should try to support the child in a head downwards position (Figure 3.20). If the child is too large to do this safely, they should be supported in a forward-leaning position, with the rescuer delivering the back blows from behind.

2. Up to 5 sharp blows should be delivered to the middle of the child's back, between their scapulae, with the heel of the rescuer's other hand.

The aim is to relieve the obstruction with each individual back blow rather than to give all 5.

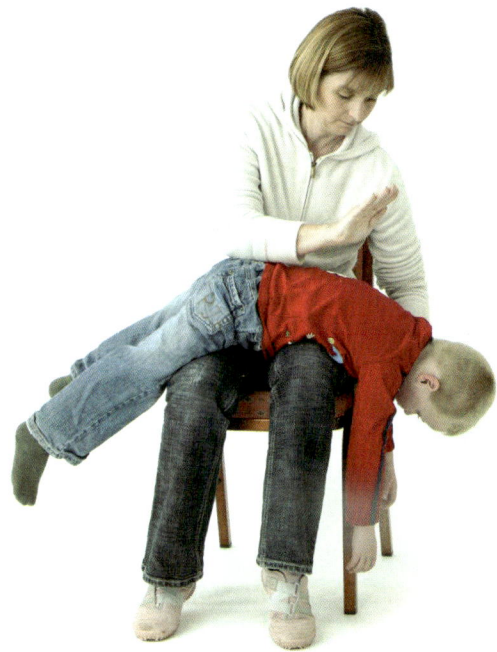

Figure 3.20 Delivery of back blows to a child

If back blows fail to dislodge the foreign body and the infant/child is still conscious, the rescuer should give *thrusts*. In infants these are delivered to the chest, and are similar to chest compressions. However, in children over one year, abdominal thrusts may be performed. If the clinical judgement of the rescuer is that the child is too small to tolerate abdominal thrusts, then chest thrusts can be delivered instead. **Abdominal thrusts (Heimlich manoeuvre) must not be performed on infants.**

Delivery of chest thrusts to an infant

1. The rescuer should turn the infant from the head downwards, prone position they were in for back blow delivery, into a head downwards, supine position. This can be safely achieved by placement of the rescuer's free arm along the infant's back, with the hand encircling the infant's occiput. The infant should then be turned over whilst keeping their head lower than their trunk.

2. The rescuer must support the infant down their arm which is supported down (or across) their thigh.

3. The landmark for chest compressions (Figures 3.12 and 3.13) should be identified on the infant's sternum and up to 5 sharp downward thrusts delivered. These thrusts are similar to chest compressions but they are sharper in nature and delivered at a slower rate.

The aim is to relieve the obstruction with each individual chest thrust rather than to give all 5.

Delivery of abdominal thrusts to a child over one year

1. To maximise safety, the rescuer should stand behind the child, and support them in a forward leaning position by placing their arms underneath the child's and encircling their torso.

2. The rescuer should clench one of their fists and place it against the child's abdomen, approximately midway between the umbilicus and the xiphisternum.

3. By grasping their fist with their free hand, the rescuer should give the abdominal thrusts by pulling sharply inwards and upwards up to 5 times (Figure 3.21). Care should be taken not to exert pressure over the xiphoid process or the lower rib cage as this may result in thoracic or intra-abdominal trauma.

The aim is to relieve the obstruction with each individual abdominal thrust rather than to give all 5.

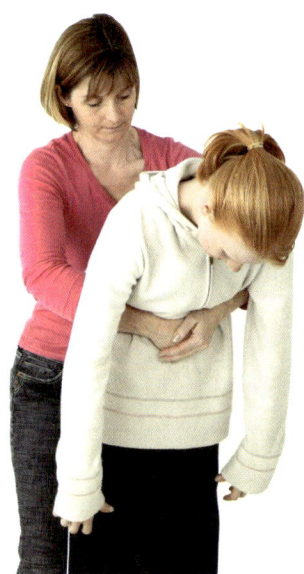

Figure 3.21 Delivery of abdominal thrusts to a child

Reassessment

Following delivery of the chest or abdominal thrusts, the rescuer must reassess the child.

If the foreign body has been successfully expelled, the child may still need medical assistance; a piece of the object may remain in the respiratory tract and cause further complications. As abdominal thrusts can cause injury, a child who has received them should be examined by a medical practitioner.

If the foreign body has not been expelled and the child remains conscious, repeat the sequence of back blows and thrusts as indicated. Do not leave the child at this stage, but call out again to ensure that the EMS has been called.

Unresponsive infants and children

If the child is, or becomes, unconscious from choking, they should be placed supine on a firm, flat surface, whilst the rescuer shouts for help. If, a second rescuer is available, they should be sent to activate the EMS. If there is only one rescuer, they must not leave the child at this stage, but proceed with BLS as described earlier in this chapter, with particular attention to the following points:

Checking the mouth

Each time the airway is opened for rescue breaths, the rescuer should look to see if they can detect the foreign body in the child's mouth. If it is visible, a single finger sweep can be attempted to remove the object. However, blind or repeated finger sweeps must not be performed as these are likely to impact the object further down the pharynx and/or cause trauma.

Initial rescue breaths

When a rescue breath attempt does not result in chest wall expansion, the child's head should be repositioned before attempting the next breath. If, despite repositioning, all 5 rescue breaths are ineffective and the child remains unresponsive (no 'signs of life'), the rescuer should proceed straight to chest compressions.

Continued BLS

The sequence of BLS should be followed with a check for the foreign body in the child's mouth made before attempting the 2 rescue breaths. If the first rescue breath is ineffective, the head should be repositioned before attempting the second. If the second is also ineffective, the rescuer should proceed with chest compressions.

If rescue breaths are effective at making the chest rise, the rescuer should continue full BLS until the child shows signs of life.

If the child displays signs of life, the rescuer should assess their ABC and continue as appropriate.

Recovery positions

Unless contraindicated, the unresponsive child who has effective spontaneous breathing should be placed in a safe side-lying position (Figure 3.22).

The purpose of placing an unresponsive child in such a position is to ensure that their tongue does not fall backwards occluding their pharynx, and to reduce the potential risk of aspiration should they vomit.

There is no universally accepted 'recovery' position for children, but there are general principles to be considered when placing the child in a safe position. These include ensuring that the child:

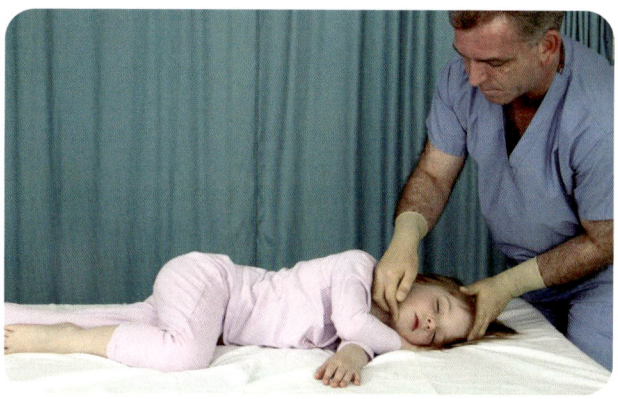

Figure 3.22 An unresponsive child in a safe side-lying position

- has a patent airway
- can drain secretions/vomit freely from their mouth
- is in a stable position that they cannot easily roll over from (this may require the placement of a rolled-up towel or blanket behind their back in small infants)
- can be easily observed
- can be easily turned on to their back if they require resuscitation interventions
- is in as near a true lateral position as possible
- has no pressure on their chest that may impede breathing

If the child needs to be in this position for longer than an hour, they should be turned on to their other side to relieve the pressure on the lower arm.

Key learning points

- **Rescuers must always ensure their own safety before undertaking BLS**
- **The preferred ratio of chest compressions: ventilations is 15:2 when BLS is being delivered by healthcare professionals but in some instances it may be appropriate to adopt the standard adult 30:2 sequence**
- **One full minute of BLS should be performed by lone rescuers before they activate EMS (except on the rare occasion that a primary cardiac arrest is suspected)**
- **Management of conscious choking infants consists of back blows followed by chest thrusts**
- **Management of conscious choking children consists of back blows followed by abdominal thrusts**
- **Management of unconscious infants and children with choking requires BLS to be performed**

EUROPEAN PAEDIATRIC LIFE SUPPORT

Further reading

Atkins DL, Everson-Stewart S, Sears GK, Daya M, Osmond MH, Warden CR, et al. Epidemiology and outcomes from out-of-hospital cardiac arrest in children: the Resuscitation Outcomes Consortium Epistry-Cardiac Arrest. Circulation. 2009 Mar 24;119(11):1484-91.

Nadkarni VM, Larkin GL, Peberdy MA, Carey SM, Kaye W, Mancini ME, et al. First documented rhythm and clinical outcome from in-hospital cardiac arrest among children and adults. JAMA. 2006 Jan 4;295(1):50-7.

Kitamura T, Iwami T, Kawamura T, Nagao K, Tanaka H, Nadkarni VM, et al. Conventional and chest-compression-only cardiopulmonary resuscitation by bystanders for children who have out-of-hospital cardiac arrests: a prospective, nationwide, population-based cohort study. Lancet. 2010 Apr 17;375(9723):1347-54.

Kao PC, Chiang WC, Yang CW, Chen SJ, Liu YP, Lee CC, et al. What is the correct depth of chest compression for infants and children? A radiological study. Pediatrics. 2009 Jul;124(1):49-55.

Meyer A, Nadkarni V, Pollock A, Babbs C, Nishisaki A, Braga M, et al. Evaluation of the Neonatal Resuscitation Program's recommended chest compression depth using computerized tomography imaging. Resuscitation. 2010 May;81(5):544-8.

Sutton RM, Niles D, Nysaether J, Arbogast KB, Nishisaki A, Maltese MR, et al. Pediatric CPR quality monitoring: analysis of thoracic anthropometric data. Resuscitation. 2009 Oct;80(10):1137-41.

Babbs SF, Nadkarni V. Optimizing chest compression to rescue ventilation ratios during one-rescue CPR by professionals and laypersons: children are not just little adults. Resuscitation 2004; 61:173-81.

Berg RA, Hilwig RW et al. "Simulated mouth-to-mouth ventilation and chest compressions (bystander cardiopulmonary resuscitation) improves outcome in a swine model of prehospital pediatric asphyxial cardiac arrest." Crit Care Med 1999; 27(9):1893-1899.

Berg RA, Hilwig RW et al. "Bystander" chest compressions and assisted ventilation independently improve outcome from piglet asphyxial pulseless "cardiac arrest". Circulation 2000; 101(14):1743-1748.

Tibballs J, Russell P. Reliability of pulse palpation by healthcare personnel to diagnose paediatric cardiac arrest. Resuscitation. 2009 Jan;80(1):61-4.

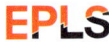

Advanced Management of the Airway and Ventilation

CHAPTER 4

Learning outcomes

To understand:

- How to recognise upper airway obstruction
- The methods used to open the airway during initial resuscitation
- How to use oxygen delivery systems during initial resuscitation
- The methods used to assist ventilation during initial resuscitation
- The role of advanced airways (laryngeal masks and tracheal tubes) during initial resuscitation

LOOK for chest (and abdominal) movements

LISTEN for airflow at the mouth and nose (+/- additional noises)

FEEL for airflow at the mouth and nose

As previously described, the most common cause of cardiorespiratory arrest in children is secondary to respiratory failure resulting in hypoxia and acidosis. The outcome is poor following hypoxic induced cardiorespiratory arrest therefore the management of the airway and ventilation (breathing) is the first priority in dealing with the seriously ill child regardless of the underlying cause. Early recognition and adequate management of compensated respiratory failure are therefore essential. This chapter describes the initial advanced management of the airway and ventilation based on the child's physiological dysfunction.

Airway obstruction

Airway obstruction is a common occurrence in the seriously ill child. It may be the primary cause of the cardiorespiratory arrest (e.g. choking) or a consequence of the underlying disease process (i.e. hypoxia), which leads to loss of consciousness. In the unconscious child, the tongue can fall backwards and occlude their airway (Figure 4.1). Regardless of the cause, airway obstruction must be rapidly recognised and managed to prevent secondary hypoxic damage to the vital organs.

Recognition of airway obstruction

In a conscious child, airway obstruction may be demonstrated by difficulty in breathing and/or increased respiratory effort. In both conscious and unconscious children, there may be additional respiratory noises if the obstruction is partial, whereas respiration will be silent if there is complete obstruction.

The most effective way to detect airway obstruction in all children is to look, listen and feel.

LOOK for breathing – during normal breathing, the chest wall expands and the abdomen is pushed slightly outwards as the diaphragm contracts. When the airway is obstructed however, the abdomen protrudes markedly and the chest is drawn inwards when the diaphragm contracts during inspiration ('see-saw' respiration). Additionally, accessory muscle usage and recession are likely to be observed. It can be difficult to differentiate these paradoxical movements from normal breathing, and it is therefore essential to also listen for the presence or absence of breath sounds and feel for air movement. If a clear face mask is being used, misting of the mask may be observed.

LISTEN for breathing – normal respiration is quiet. Partially obstructed breathing is noisy, whilst completely obstructed breathing will be silent.

FEEL for breathing – the movement of air on inspiration and expiration can be felt at the mouth and nose (or tracheostomy) during normal breathing. If there is airway obstruction this will be limited or absent.

Partial airway obstruction can quickly deteriorate to complete obstruction and therefore must always be considered as an emergency. Complete airway obstruction will lead to profound hypoxia, vital organ failure and cardiorespiratory arrest if the obstruction is not relieved very rapidly. Immediate action must be taken to relieve the obstruction and clear the airway.

Techniques to optimise the airway

Conscious children

If the child is making adequate spontaneous respiratory effort, they should be supported in a position of comfort (preferably the one they naturally assume themselves to optimise their airway). High-flow oxygen should be given in a manner that the child will tolerate, whilst experienced help is sought.

Unconscious children

Whether or not the child is making spontaneous respiratory effort, the patency of the airway needs to be optimised immediately. This initially means positioning their head by performing either a head tilt and chin lift, or a jaw thrust manoeuvre. Additionally, suction may be required to clear secretions, vomit or blood.

Head positioning

The rescuer can open the child's airway by performing a head tilt and chin lift (Figure 4.2) or jaw thrust manoeuvre (Chapter 3). It is extremely important to ensure that head positioning techniques are carried out properly to make certain that neither hyperextension (Figure 4.3) nor excessive flexion of the neck occurs, as both will make obstruction worse. The rescuer must also take care not to compress the soft tissues under the child's jaw as this can also occlude the airway.

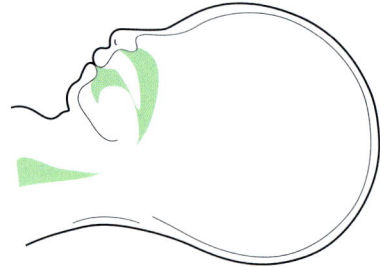

Figure 4.1 Unconscious child, the tongue falls backwards and obstructs the airway

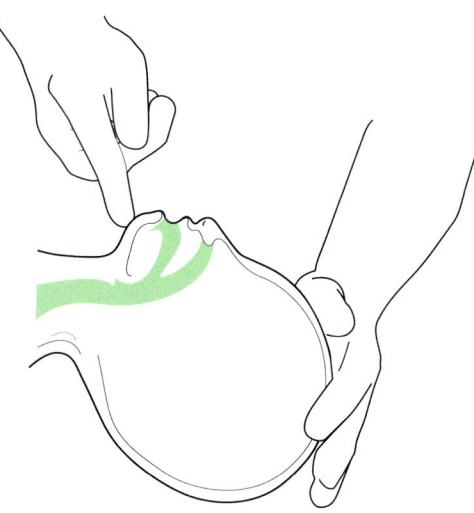

Figure 4.2 Head tilt chin lift opens the airway

Suction

Standard suction devices in hospital are pipeline units. They consist of a wall terminal outlet, vacuum pressure regulator, a reservoir, tubing and a connector for an appropriate suction catheter to be attached.

In some low dependency hospital areas, during transportation and non-hospital environments such as GP surgeries, it is likely that the suction device available will be a portable device that is operated by battery or a hand/foot pump.

Large bore rigid suction catheters (e.g. Yankauer) are particularly useful for the clearance of thick or excessive secretions and vomit. Soft, flexible catheters in a range of sizes should also be available as these may be less traumatic to use and are particularly useful for nasal suction. They can also be passed through nasopharyngeal or oropharyngeal airways and tracheal tubes but they may not allow adequate clearance of thick or copious secretions.

Whichever suction catheter types are used, they should ideally have a side hole that can be occluded by the rescuer's finger to allow greater control over the suction pressure generated. Suction pressure should not exceed 120 mmHg in infants.

Airway suction must be carried out cautiously if the child has an intact gag reflex as it may induce vomiting which can lead to aspiration.

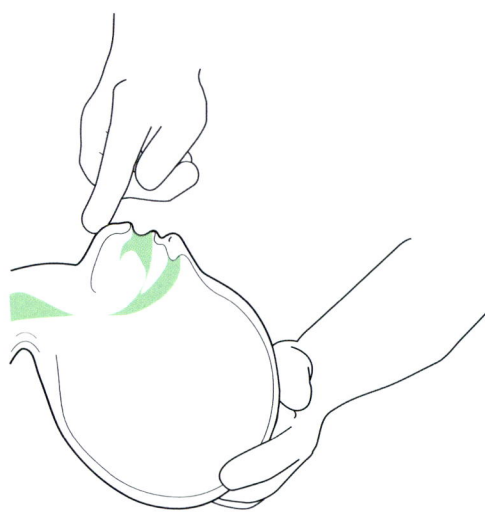

Figure 4.3 Hyperextension obstructs the airway

Airway opening adjuncts

Oropharyngeal airways

The oropharyngeal airway (e.g. Guedel) is a rigid curved tube that is designed to open a channel between the lips and the base of the tongue (Figure 4.4). They are made of plastic and are reinforced and flanged at the proximal end. Available sizes range from 000 for premature infants to 4-5 for large adults (Figure 4.5).

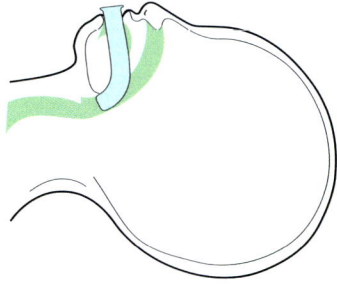

Figure 4.4 Airway adjunct keeps the tongue forward

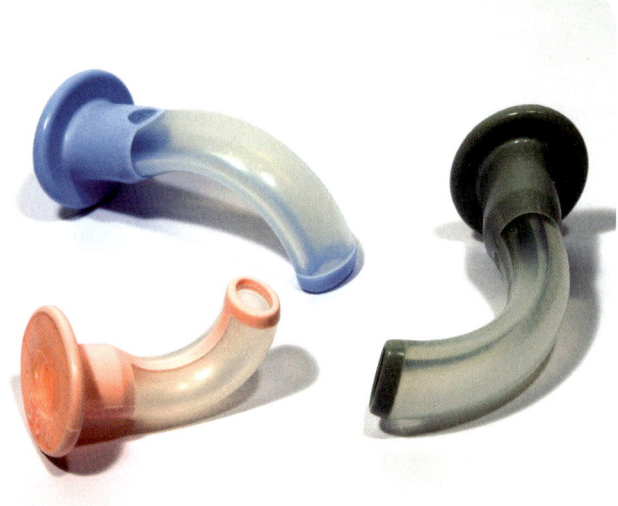

Figure 4.5 Oropharyngeal airways

The correctly sized airway is one that, when laid against the side of the face, has a length equal to the distance between the level of the patient's incisors (or where they will be) to the angle of their jaw (Figure 4.6). If an incorrect size is used, it may result in trauma, laryngospasm and/or worsening of the airway obstruction.

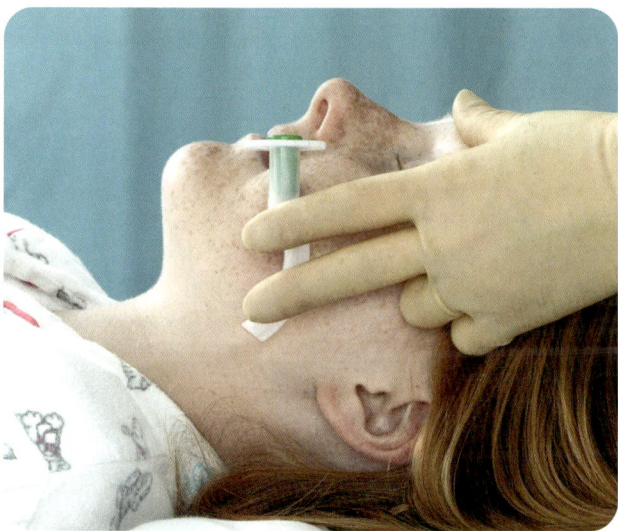

Figure 4.6 Measuring the appropriate oropharyngeal airway in a child

The oropharyngeal airway should be inserted with great care using the minimum of force to avoid trauma and bleeding of the delicate palatal and pharyngeal mucosa. It is important to ensure that the tip of the oropharyngeal airway does not push the tongue back into the pharynx.

The airway can be introduced directly, sliding it carefully over the tongue or alternatively, it can be introduced upside down initially, as follows:

- place the tip with the concave side of the airway facing the roof of the mouth

- insert the airway past the teeth and gums pushing the tongue away from the roof of the mouth with the convex side of the airway

- rotate it 180° as it passes beyond the hard palate and into the oropharynx

- ensure that the flange rest over the mouth

Whichever technique is used, the effort required to insert the oropharyngeal airway should be minimal; **do not use force!**

Oropharyngeal airways are intended to be used only in unconscious patients. If the child is semi-conscious they may cough, gag, vomit or develop laryngospasm. Insertion of the oropharyngeal airway should be abandoned if this occurs.

Following insertion of the oropharyngeal airway, the child's airway patency should be reassessed by the 'look, listen and feel' approach and oxygen given if indicated.

Nasopharyngeal airways

The nasopharyngeal airway is a flexible tube that is designed to open a channel between the nostril and the nasopharynx. They are made of soft plastic or silicone, are bevelled at the insertion end and flanged at the outer end (Figure 4.7). To prevent them passing completely into the nostril, the proximal end should have a large flange or a safety pin can be fastened through the end of the tube. Tracheal tubes cut to the correct length may be used instead.

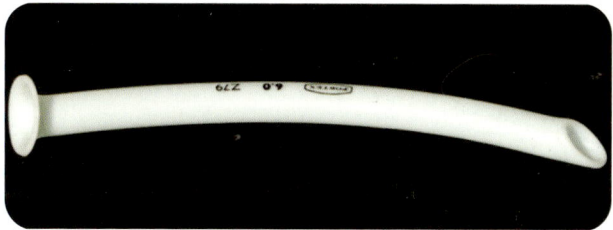

Figure 4.7 Nasopharyngeal airway

The correctly sized nasopharyngeal airway is estimated by measuring the distance from the tip of the child's nostril to the tragus of the ear. An appropriate tube size can be estimated by matching its diameter against the diameter of the child's anterior nares and when inserted it should not cause blanching of the nostril.

Once appropriately sized, the nasopharyngeal airway should be lubricated and introduced into the nostril. With a gentle rotating motion, the airway should be passed directly backwards and posteriorly along the floor of the nostril. The tube should not be directed upwards as this will cause trauma and bleeding (Figure 4.8).

Nasopharyngeal airways may be better tolerated by conscious children than oropharyngeal airways and are useful as adjuncts in the management of children who may improve their level of consciousness, e.g. the fitting child who is becoming less obtunded.

Their use is contraindicated in patients where basal skull fracture is suspected or if there is a coagulopathy.

EUROPEAN PAEDIATRIC LIFE SUPPORT

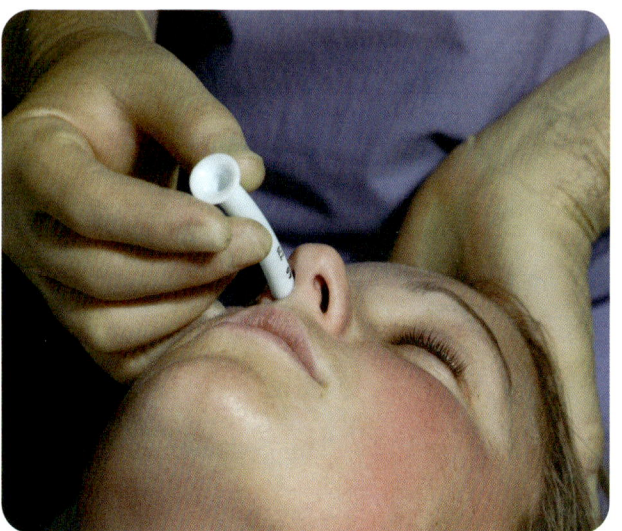

Figure 4.8 Insertion of a nasopharyngeal airway

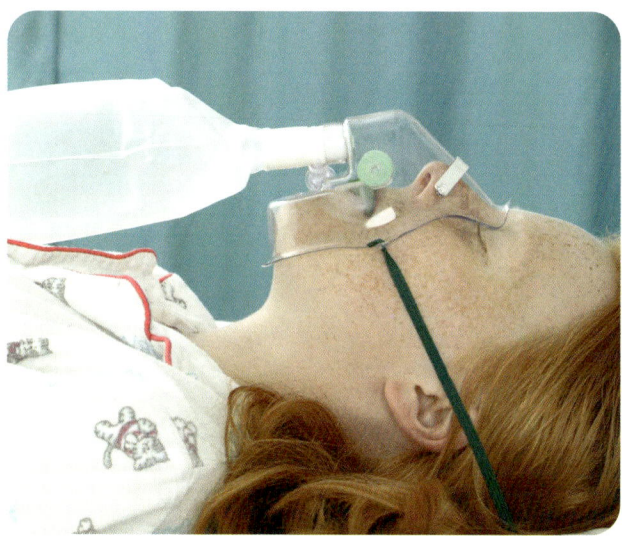

Figure 4.9 Non re-breathing oxygen mask with reservoir

Following insertion of the nasopharyngeal airway, the child's airway patency should be reassessed by the 'look, listen and feel' approach and oxygen given if indicated.

Oxygen delivery systems

Oxygen should be given as soon as it is available. Initially, this should be at the highest available concentration for all seriously ill children; concerns about oxygen toxicity should never prevent its use during resuscitation. Oxygen should be regulated using a flowmeter capable of delivering up to 15 l min^{-1}. It should ideally be warmed and humidified to minimise the risks of airway irritation and hypothermia. The method used to deliver the oxygen should be selected according to the child's clinical condition. Oxygen saturation levels should be monitored by pulse oximetry (SpO$_2$). When the child's condition has stabilised, the inspired oxygen concentration should be reduced, whilst monitoring SpO$_2$ to maintain adequate oxygenation.

Oxygen mask with reservoir bag

This is the preferred method for delivering oxygen in the seriously ill child who is breathing spontaneously. The flow of oxygen must be sufficiently high to ensure the reservoir bag fills adequately (Figure 4.9). It is possible to give an oxygen concentration up to 90% with an oxygen delivery flow of 12-15 l min^{-1} depending on the child's minute volume (the product of the tidal volume of each breath and the number of breaths per minute).

These devices have three 'one-way' flap-valves; one between the oxygen supply port/reservoir bag and the mask, and one on each side of the facemask over the inspiratory holes.

The mask works as follows:

- when the child inhales, the valve between oxygen supply port/reservoir bag and the mask opens allowing oxygen to flow in to the mask, whilst the ones on either side of the mask close so reducing entrainment of room air, hence minimising the dilution of the higher concentration of inspired oxygen.

- when the child exhales, the valve between oxygen supply port/reservoir bag and the mask closes whilst the ones on either side of the mask opens to allow escape of the child's expired breath (i.e. there is no rebreathing of gas).

Note: if the flap-valves are inadvertently removed, re-breathing and dilution of inspired oxygen can occur.

Simple oxygen mask

A simple oxygen mask without a reservoir bag can deliver oxygen concentrations of up to 60% at flow rates of 10-15 l min^{-1}. Room air is entrained around the edges of the mask and through the holes in the mask so diluting the oxygen delivery.

'Blow-by' facial oxygen

Either the end of the oxygen tubing or a facemask can be held by the child's carer at a short distance from the child's face. This is a less-threatening method that can help to alleviate the child's fear and maximise their cooperation. However, the inspired concentration that can be delivered is low and inconsistent, so it is only suitable for children with mild respiratory compromise who cannot tolerate other methods of oxygen delivery. Oxygen flow rates need to be adjusted depending what the child will accept.

Headbox oxygen

This method may be useful in small infants. It permits reliable measurement and control of the inspired oxygen (FiO$_2$) level, as well as allowing warming and humidification of the delivered oxygen. However, the FiO$_2$ rapidly falls when the lid is removed from the headbox to undertake care procedures or a full assessment of the infant's clinical condition. Rapid access to the infant's head can be difficult, and therefore headbox oxygen delivery is not appropriate during resuscitation.

Nasal cannulae

This method can be useful in stable children of all ages, particularly in pre-school children. The delivery of oxygen via cannulae (or 'prongs') is dependent on oxygen flow and nasal resistance but the FiO_2 will be low and variable, so it is not suitable during resuscitation or when a high oxygen concentration is required. Flow rates should be kept below 3 l min^{-1} as higher flows are extremely irritating to the nasal passages and do not significantly increase oxygen delivery. Nasal cannulae are not suitable for use in children with copious or tenacious nasal secretions, as the cannulae will be easily blocked.

Methods of assisted ventilation

When providing positive pressure ventilation for an infant/child, the rescuer should aim for a respiratory rate of 12-20 min^{-1} with younger children having higher rates. In a newborn the rate should be 30 min^{-1}. The volume delivered should be sufficient to produce a normal visible chest expansion and breath sounds on auscultation. Continuous monitoring of the heart rate and SpO_2 should be undertaken as soon as practicable.

Mouth-to-mask devices

Rescuers should not delay giving rescue breaths until the arrival of advanced paediatric airway and ventilation equipment, and therefore expired air breaths (e.g. mouth-to-mouth) using a barrier device such as a face shield may be more appropriate in initial resuscitation attempts.

The pocket mask is widely used in resuscitation of apnoeic adults and the standard size may be suitable for use in larger children and adolescents. There is a 'paediatric' pocket mask available but it should be noted that this one size does not fit all infants and children, and an appropriate size of paediatric facemask may need to be substituted. Expired air ventilation using pocket mask should only be used if a manual ventilation device (e.g. self-inflating bag system) is not immediately available.

When it is deemed appropriate for use (e.g. in an adolescent) the pocket mask is a device designed to minimise infection risks when delivering expired air ventilation. The device is made of transparent plastic with a one-way valve that directs the patient's expired breath away from the rescuer. An oxygen delivery port (which also has a one-way valve) is incorporated into some pocket masks and allows supplemental oxygen to be administered.

Technique for mouth-to-mask ventilation:

- Having assembled the pocket mask, the rescuer positions themselves behind the supine child

- The child's head should be placed in an appropriate position (e.g. 'sniffing' position) to achieve a patent airway

- Apply the mask over the child's mouth and nose, pressing down with the thumbs of both hands to create a seal

- Lift the child's jaw upwards (jaw thrust) into the mask with the other fingers, taking care not to compress the soft tissues under the mandible

- Blow through the mask's one-way valve until chest expansion is observed (Figure 4.10)

- Stop inflation and observe the chest falling

- Repeat as appropriate

- If chest expansion is not seen, assess whether this may be due to inadequate airway patency or a poor seal between the child's face and the mask, and correct as necessary

- If the mask has an appropriate port and there is oxygen available, supplemental oxygen should be administered

This technique can also be used with a standard facemask, but it will not provide protection against infection unless a breathing system filter is also used.

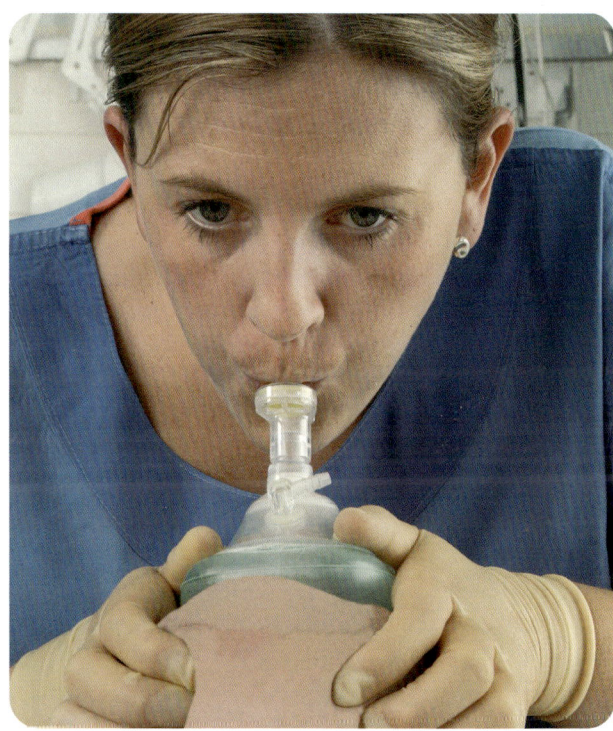

Figure 4.10 Ventilation with a pocket mask

The self-inflating bag device (as used for bag-mask ventilation)

In a child who has inadequate/absent breathing, maintenance of a patent airway is the first priority of management. Once this is achieved, adequate ventilation must be established. The self-inflating bag system with an oxygen reservoir is the first line system for providing ventilation during resuscitation. Although the self-inflating bag can be used without a supplemental oxygen source, in resuscitation situations it is usually used to deliver ventilation with high-flow oxygen. The self-inflating bag can be connected not only to a facemask but also to a tracheal tube or laryngeal mask airway when these are in place.

The self-inflating bag operates in the following manner:

Inspiration – squeezing of the bag by the rescuer allows oxygen enriched air to flow through a one way inspiratory (non-rebreathing) valve at the patient end of the device and hence to the patient. A valve at the oxygen port/reservoir end of the system prevents gases entering the reservoir bag.

Expiration – when the squeezing pressure on the bag is stopped, passively expired gases from the patient pass out into the atmosphere through the non-rebreathing valve at the patient end of the device. The bag reinflates, owing to its elastic recoil, and oxygen enters the bag via the oxygen port and via the reservoir bag so increasing the oxygen concentration in the bag.

Used without supplemental oxygen, a self-inflating bag system will ventilate with room air (21% oxygen). The oxygen concentration can be increased to approximately 50% by attaching a high flow of oxygen to the oxygen port on the base of the bag, without a reservoir bag. The use of the reservoir bag, as described above together with high-flow of oxygen at 15 l min^{-1}, will enable the delivery of > 90% oxygen (Figure 4.11).

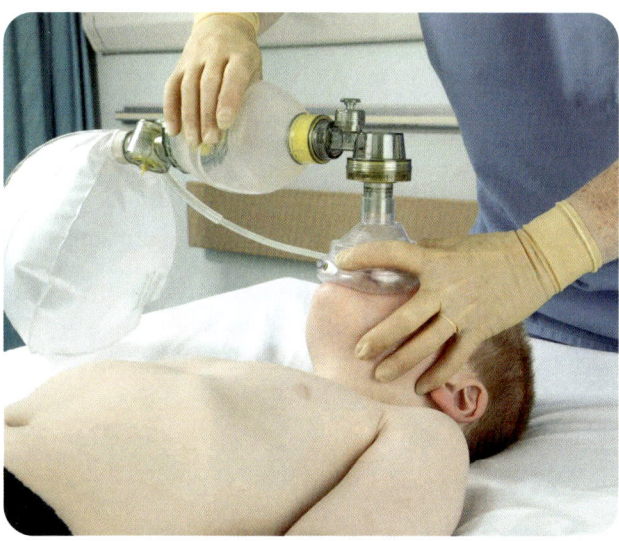

Figure 4.11 Ventilation of a child with a self-inflating bag-mask device

Self-inflating bags are available in four sizes (generally 250, 450-500, 900-1200 and 1600-2000 ml). The two smallest sizes usually have a pressure-limiting valve that prevents excessive inflation pressures that otherwise may cause barotrauma. The pressure limit is pre-determined by the manufacturers (usually 30-40 cmH$_2$O). During resuscitation, higher than normal inflation pressures may be required and the pressure limiting valve may need to be over-ridden. The most common cause of needing to activate the pressure-limiting valve is upper airway obstruction due to a poor airway opening technique. Thus ensure that the child's airway is patent (e.g. check head positioning) before overriding the valve. It should be noted that such valves are now being incorporated into some of the large bag sizes.

The smallest bag (250 ml) is intended for use in preterm neonates < 2.5 kg only. It is not appropriate for use in full term neonates and infants as it may be inadequate to support effective tidal volume.

The second size of bag (450-500 ml) is generally most appropriate for full term neonates, infants and pre-schoolchildren. Many paediatric hospitals will also stock the 900 to 1200 ml size bags for school age children/early adolescence as the largest size (1600 to 2000 ml) can be more unwieldy to use. Regardless of size the provider should only use the force and tidal volume necessary to cause visible chest expansion. (Figures 4.11, 4.12).

Self-inflating bags should not be used to deliver oxygen to spontaneously breathing patients. Depending on the valve system, this may result in the inspiration of room air (or even rebreathing of the child's own passively expired air if the mask is held tightly on the face) as the child's own respiratory efforts may not generate sufficient pressure to open the valve. Children, who are making adequate respiratory effort, should therefore have oxygen administered by another method.

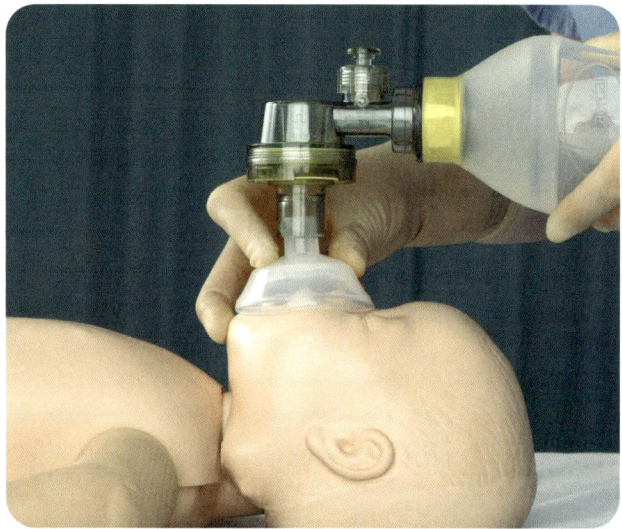

Figure 4.12 Ventilation of an infant with a self-inflating bag-mask device

Facemask selection

These are the interface between the ventilation device and the child. They must be capable of providing a good seal over the mouth and nose whilst ensuring minimal pressure is applied over the eyes.

Masks are available in a variety of sizes and two basic types; anatomically shaped ones for older children and adults, and circular ones for infants and small children (Figure 4.13). The preferred mask is transparent (to allow rapid detection of secretions/vomit and observation of the child's central colour) and should have a low dead space.

Bag-mask ventilation

Ventilatory support using assisted ventilation is indicated in the child with decompensated respiratory failure. Bag-mask ventilation (BMV) describes the use of a facemask and a self-inflating bag system with an oxygen reservoir attached that delivers positive pressure ventilation without rebreathing of expired respiratory gases, as described above.

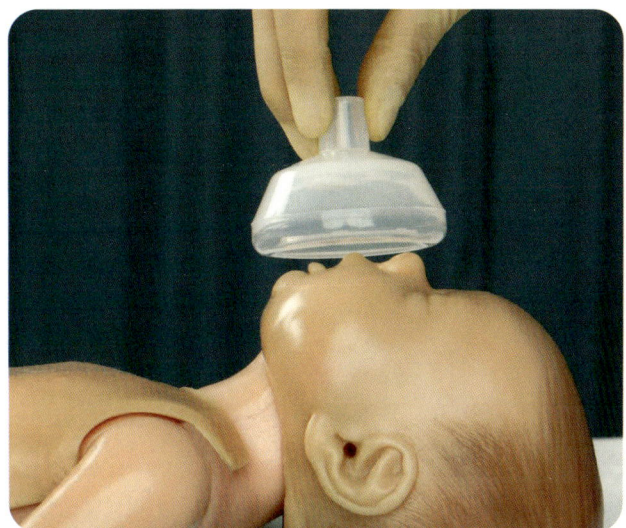

Figure 4.13 Selection of facemask for an infant

Correctly performed BMV is an essential skill for all healthcare professionals who work with children. Whilst the operating principle of self-inflating bags is simple, they require skill to use them safely and effectively.

Hypoventilation can occur with poor technique (e.g. inadequate mask seal or incorrect head positioning) and is likely to have a negative effect on outcome.

Excessive ventilation volume can distend the stomach which reduces ventilation by limiting the movement of the diaphragm and increases the risk of gastro-oesophageal reflux and the aspiration of gastric contents.

When self-inflating bags are used with a facemask, it can be difficult for a single rescuer to achieve an airtight seal whilst simultaneously using one hand to maintain a patent airway with a jaw thrust manoeuvre, and squeezing the bag with the other. A two-person technique (one person to maintain the airway and hold the mask in position, and the second to squeeze the bag) will usually overcome these difficulties (Figure 4.14).

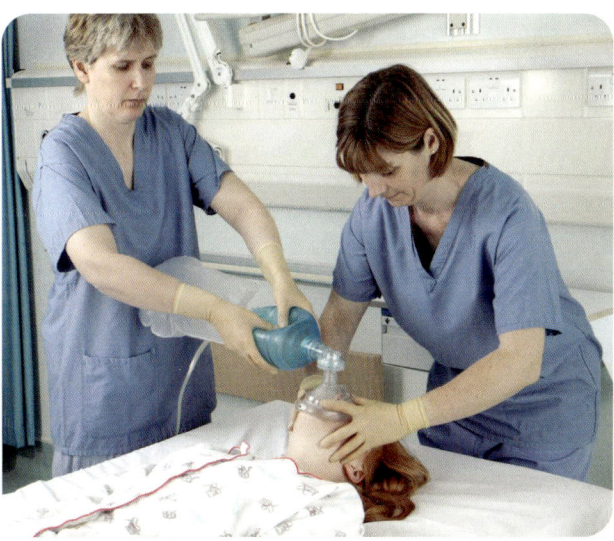

Figure 4.14 Self-inflating bag-mask device in use by two rescuers on a child

Technique for bag-mask ventilation

- Having selected the appropriate size of bag and mask, the rescuer should stand behind the supine child

- The oxygen supply should be connected at a high flow and the reservoir bag should be seen to inflate

- If there is a second person available they should stand at one side of the child

- The child's head should be placed in an appropriate position (e.g. 'neutral' position for an infant, 'sniffing the morning air' in the older child) to achieve a patent airway. A roll placed under the infant's shoulders is often useful to assist in maintaining an appropriate airway position (unless contraindicated in trauma cases)

- Apply the mask over the child's mouth and nose, gently pressing down with the thumb and index finger of one hand (or both hands if two rescuers)

- Lift the child's jaw upwards (jaw thrust) into the mask with the other fingers, with one finger under the angle of the jaw. Take care not to compress the soft tissues underneath the mandible

- Gently squeeze the bag until chest expansion is observed to a normal chest expansion

- Stop inflation and observe the chest falling

- Repeat as appropriate

- If chest expansion is not seen, assess whether this may be due to inadequate airway patency or a poor seal between the child's face and the mask, and correct as necessary

Bag-mask ventilation frequently results in gastric distension, and therefore placement of a gastric tube should be undertaken as early as practicable.

T-piece (flow-inflating bag) circuit

This equipment is often employed by anaesthesia or ICU staff. It requires a continuous gas source for inflation of the bag, and therefore there must always be an appropriate self-inflating system immediately available, in case there is a failure of the gas supply. This circuit does not have any valves and the bag has an open end. To achieve ventilation the end of the bag needs to be occluded and the bag squeezed. To prevent rebreathing a high gas flow is required (at least three times the minute ventilation of the patient, i.e. > 30 ml kg^{-1} × respiratory rate). This circuit can deliver 100% oxygen and can be used in spontaneously breathing children. The bag of this device gives some 'feeling' of the compliance of the lungs and allows some positive end expiratory pressure (PEEP) to be applied manually. The safe and effective use of this equipment requires considerable expertise and it should be utilised by experienced practitioners only.

Supraglottic upper airway devices:

Laryngeal mask airway (LMA)

The LMA is a supraglottic airway device, which is widely used in children undergoing routine surgical procedures as a means of providing an effective airway to achieve ventilation and oxygenation (Figure 4.15). Like the oropharyngeal airway, it can cause gagging, coughing and laryngospasm in children who are semi-conscious, so it should only be used in unconscious patients with relaxed jaw muscles.

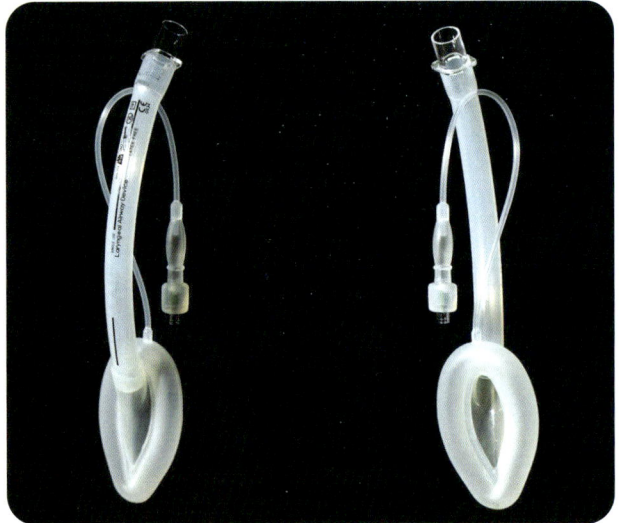

Figure 4.15 Laryngeal mask airway

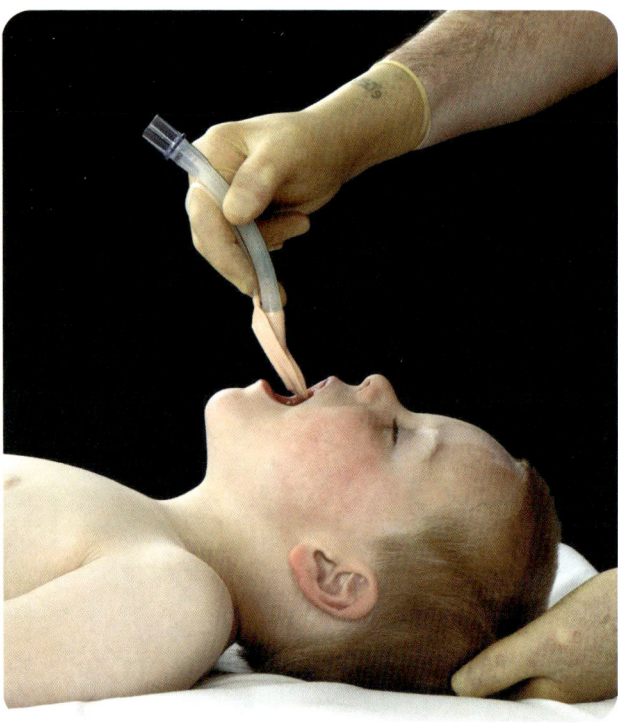

Figure 4.16 Insertion of laryngeal mask airway

LMA insertion should be considered by trained providers if BMV is not successful. It is an alternative to tracheal intubation when suitably skilled individuals are not available.

It consists of a tube with an inflatable cuffed mask at the distal end, which is introduced into the mouth and advanced into the pharynx, until resistance is felt (Figure 4.16). The cuff is then inflated, providing a low pressure seal over the laryngeal inlet. This leaves the distal opening of the tube just above the vocal cords. The LMA does not protect the lungs from regurgitation and aspiration of gastric contents.

Recent evidence has shown that, in situations when BMV is not successful as a first line method of oxygenation and ventilation, the LMA may be a useful alternative, provided the healthcare professional has had appropriate training in its use.

LMA insertion technique

The correct size of LMA is based on the age of the child (Table 4.1). The LMA can be either sterilized reusable or single use. Prior to insertion the device should be inspected for damage and tubing obstruction. The cuff should be checked for leaks by inflation to 50% greater than the recommended inflation volume. A water soluble lubricant gel needs to be applied to the tip and back of the cuff, just before insertion.

There have been several methods described to insert the LMA in children. In general it is useful to consider the LMA as slightly longer oropharyngeal airway with the distal cuff sitting over the laryngeal inlet.

The following is the standard insertion technique:

- the cuff is fully deflated and the tubing is held by the dominant hand of the rescuer, just above the cuff (Figure 4.16)

- whilst standing behind the child's head, the other hand holds the occiput and gently extends the head

- the tip of the mask is inserted into the child's mouth and is pressed against the hard palate

- the mask is advanced into the mouth until the cuff passes beyond the back of the tongue. Stop pushing the mask once resistance is felt (the cuff should not be visible in the mouth once the mask is in place)

- once the LMA is correctly positioned, the cuff should be slowly inflated using an air filled syringe. (Table 4.1)

- a small outward movement of the tube is frequently seen once the correct volume is given, this is the moment to stop inflating the cuff

- the opening of the cuff must facing forward once the LMA is inserted to lie above the laryngeal inlet, i.e. towards the patient's feet

- a self-inflating bag system is connected to the LMA and gentle squeezed. The chest should be seen to rise in a similar manner to that when performing BMV

- the LMA should be secured in place using tape.

If resistance is felt while attempting to pass the cuff beyond the back of the tongue, various strategies can be used to aid insertion. The head can be further extended, the mask partially inflated and rotated 90° or 180° (like the rotation technique used to insert an oropharyngeal airway) and then further advanced. If the chest is not seen to rise the LMA should be removed and BMV should be performed.

Table 4.1 LMA size selection and cuff volume

LMA Size	Child selection	Maximum cuff volume
1	Neonates < 5 kg	4 ml
1 ½	Infants 5-10 kg	7 ml
2	Infants 10-20 kg	10 ml
2 ½	Children 20-30 kg	14 ml
3	Children 30-50 kg	20 ml

Other supraglottic airway devices

Other supraglottic airway devices for use in children (e.g. other types of LMA or laryngeal tubes) may have a role in the resuscitation of children. However, currently there is no clinical evidence to support their use.

Tracheal intubation

Tracheal intubation should only be performed by experienced personnel who have been trained to perform the technique. It is considered the "gold standard" method to achieve and maintain a secure airway. In addition, it allows optimal control of the ventilation pressures (including PEEP), prevents gastric distension, protects the lungs from aspiration of gastric contents, and makes it easier to ventilate the lungs when chest compressions are performed.

Indications

Tracheal intubation should be considered in the following situations:

- ineffective BMV
- severe anatomical or functional upper airways obstruction
- need for protection of the airway from aspiration of gastric contents
- if high pressures are required to maintain adequate oxygenation
- mechanical ventilation is required
- need for bronchial or tracheal suctioning
- instability or high probability of one of the above occurring before or during transport

Intubation can be more difficult in children compared to intubating adults. It requires extensive training, both on manikins and on real patients in the operating theatre or intensive care unit. In most situations, provided there is effective ventilation using BMV, there is no need to perform tracheal intubation until experienced personnel are available. In some circumstances e.g. head trauma and cervical spine injury, repeated attempts at intubation by the inexperienced may worsen the child's condition.

Equipment

Tracheal tubes

Traditionally uncuffed tubes have been preferred for intubation for children up to 8 years (up to 6 mm internal diameter). In these children the cricoid ring is the narrowest part of the airway and acts as a 'natural cuff'. However, recent studies have shown that there is no greater risk of complications for children between one month and 8 years when cuffed tracheal tubes are used. Consequently cuffed tracheal tubes can be considered for use in resuscitation of infants and children (except neonates) provided the correct tube size is selected, the cuff inflation pressure is monitored (20 – 25 cmH_2O) and the tube position verified. If a cuffed tracheal tube is used, the cuff should be of a high volume, low-pressure design and should be positioned below the cricoid ring, with the tracheal tube tip above the carina. Under certain circumstances (e.g. poor lung compliance, high airway resistance or a large glottic air leak) cuffed tracheal tubes have distinct advantages over uncuffed tubes.

Regardless of whether a cuffed or uncuffed tracheal tube is used, its position should be checked to ensure that the tip of the tube lies above the carina. Some tracheal tubes have markings along their length that indicate the distance the tube needs to pass, along the larynx of an average child, to rest in mid-trachea.

Choice of tracheal tube (TT)

Tube sizes are based on internal diameter (ID) in millimetres:

- **Preterm neonates:** 2.5-3.0 mm (or gestational weeks/10)
- **Term neonates:** 3.0-3.5 mm
- **Infants < 1 year:** 4.0-4.5 mm

Children over 1 year: appropriate ID is given by the formula for uncuffed TT:

$$\frac{\text{Age (years)}}{4} + 4$$

Ensure a half size larger and smaller TT are available to hand.

If a cuffed tracheal tube is used, a half size small diameter should be used.

Resuscitation tapes (e.g. Broselow, Sandell tapes) can also be used to estimate the TT size based on the child's length.

To estimate the length of TT for correct placement in the trachea, the following formulae can be used:

$$\text{Oral TT: length (cm)} = \frac{\text{Age (years)}}{2} + 12$$

or, up to 12 years, 3 x ID (cm).

$$\text{Nasal TT: length (cm)} = \frac{\text{Age (years)}}{2} + 15$$

Clinical and radiological confirmation of tube placement is essential following intubation.

Stylet

A stylet maintains the shape of TT during intubation. It must be chosen according to TT size and should be fixed so that its tip does not protrude beyond the distal end of the tube (to avoid tracheal trauma).

Laryngoscope

This consists of a body containing batteries, a light source and a blade. It must be checked prior to use and spares must always be available.

There are two types of blades; curved and straight (Figure 4.17). Their role is the same, that is, to keep the tongue out of the way and to displace the epiglottis so allowing the vocal cords to be seen.

The choice of blade type depends on personal preference and the experience of the provider, but the following age limits can act as a guide.

Straight blades (numbers 0 and 1) are usually preferred for infants (<1 year) and neonates, and are designed to lift the epiglottis under the tip of the blade so that the vocal cords can be seen. The blade may also be placed in the vallecula (between the tongue base and the epiglottis). The advantage of lifting the epiglottis is that it will then not obscure the view of the vocal cords.

Curved blades are preferred in children and adolescents (numbers 0, 1 and 2 for infants and children; 3 and 4 for adolescents and adults). They are designed to have their tip resting in the vallecula and to lift the epiglottis from above.

Straight and curved blades come in several lengths. The choice of length is guided by the child's age. If in doubt, remember that it is possible to intubate with a blade that is too long but not with one that is too short.

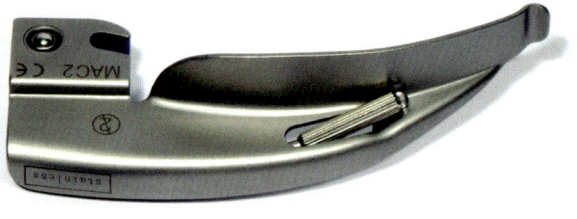
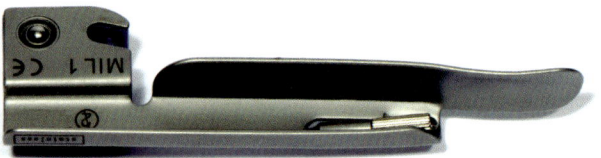

Figure 4.17 Curved and straight blades

Procedure

The ECG, heart rate and SpO_2 should be monitored during intubation. There is a risk of reflex bradycardia and hypoxia during intubation. Peripheral oxygen saturation is unreliable if peripheral perfusion is inadequate (e.g. in cardiorespiratory arrest, shock or circulatory failure).

Check all necessary equipment is available before intubation:

- Medications
- Self-inflating bag system and oxygen supply
- Oropharyngeal/nasopharyngeal airway
- Laryngoscope handles and blades
- Tracheal tubes of the appropriate sizes
- Stylet and Magill forceps
- Suction apparatus with appropriate size of suckers
- Tapes or ties to secure the tube
- Nasogastric tubes
- Capnograph (covered later in this chapter)

Intubation technique

Prior to intubation, the patient should be ventilated with 100% oxygen by BMV. If during the intubation attempt there is either a fall in peripheral oxygen saturation or bradycardia occurs, the procedure should be interrupted and the patient ventilated again with 100% oxygen by BMV.

In cardiorespiratory arrest, intubation should be performed as soon as the equipment and experienced personnel are available.

In infant <1 year, head and neck extension may be required by placing a neck roll under the shoulders (provided there is no history of cervical spine injury).

If there is suspect cervical spine injury, in-line manual immobilization of the neck should be maintained at all times during intubation.

Attempts to intubate should be interrupted if:

- The peripheral oxygen saturations reading begins to fall
- The heart rate begins to fall or is < 60 min^{-1}
- More than 30 seconds has elapsed

BMV should be recommenced until the child's condition improves before attempting intubation again.

An incorrectly placed tube or prolonged hypoxia from repeated intubation attempts can cause morbidity and even mortality.

Verification of TT placement

The position of the tube is checked by several methods as no single method is 100% reliable under all circumstances:

- Direct visualisation of the tube passing between the vocal cords
- Detect exhaled carbon dioxide via capnography
- Observe symmetrical rise of the chest
- Listen for air entry on both sides of the chest in the axillary areas
- Listen for the absence of bubbling noise over the stomach upon ventilation
- Observe for gastric distension
- Chest X-ray (after initial resuscitation)

Once the correct position is confirmed, secure TT with tape after drying and cleaning the skin with gauze.

If oesophageal intubation is suspected, remove the tube and ventilate the child by BMV or check the TT placement by direct laryngoscopy.

If auscultation is asymmetrical, and particularly if it is decreased on the left side of the chest, withdraw the TT cautiously by 0.5 cm increments until symmetrical breath sounds are heard. If breath sounds are now heard bilaterally, then the TT will have been in the right main bronchus before adjustment.

Sudden deterioration of the intubated patient

If the condition of an intubated child deteriorates, consider various possibilities, which are easily recalled by the acronym '**DOPES**':

D Displacement of the TT (accidental extubation or TT in the right main bronchus)

O Obstruction of the TT (secretions or kinking)

P Pneumothorax

E Equipment failure (check source of oxygen, ventilation bag, ventilator etc.)

S Stomach (distension can alter diaphragm mechanics)

Other reasons for deterioration or inadequate ventilation include:

- TT too small with significant air leak
- Tidal volume given too small
- Pressure-limiting valve active with non-compliant lungs (e.g. in the drowned patient)

Rapid sequence intubation (RSI)

In cardiorespiratory arrest, as the child is unconscious, intubation does not require sedation or analgesia, but in many other emergency situations both are needed.

RSI consists of the induction of anaesthesia to facilitate and secure tracheal intubation in an emergency. It reduces the incidence of adverse effects in responsive patients. These include:

- Hypoxia
- Pain
- Cardiac arrhythmias
- Rise in systemic BP and intracranial pressure
- Airway trauma
- Reflux and aspiration of gastric contents
- Psychological trauma

Oxygen must be supplied at all times. At least 3 minutes of oxygenation by BMV will provide some oxygen reserve during intubation. Atropine can be given to prevent reflex bradycardia, followed immediately by sedatives and analgesia, and by a short-acting neuromuscular blocking agent to facilitate a non-traumatic intubation.

The person performing RSI must have considerable experience in intubation and BMV, since after sedation and paralysis the child will not be able to breathe on his own. An alternative plan for airway management in case of intubation failure in RSI must have been previously considered.

Cricoid pressure (Sellick manoeuvre)

Unconscious children with a full stomach are at risk of regurgitation of gastric contents and pulmonary aspiration. The application of pressure to the cricoid cartilage occludes the oesophagus, reducing the risk of regurgitation and can be used during BMV and attempts at intubation. Cricoid pressure is difficult to perform correctly in infants and young children however, and may cause airway distortion and obstruction. **If it is thought the airway is in any way compromised, cricoid pressure should be removed immediately.**

Cricoid pressure is performed by:

- Identification of the cricoid cartilage (just below the thyroid cartilage)
- Gentle application of pressure using two fingers to the cricoid cartilage (Figure 4.19)
- The cricoid is displaced backwards to compress the oesophagus

N.B. This manoeuvre should not be performed if the child begins actively to vomit because it may lead to oesophageal rupture.

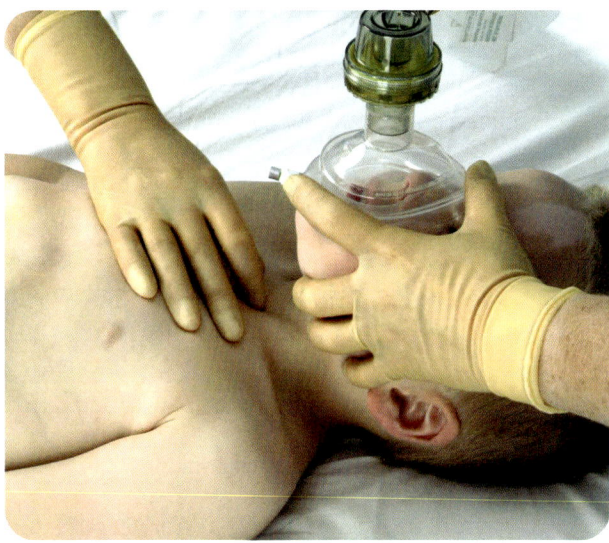

Figure 4.19 Cricoid pressure

The difficult airway

If ventilation is not possible using BMV, call for assistance and perform simple airway manoeuvres. In the majority of situations it should be possible ventilate the child until expert assistance arrives.

Occasionally, despite using these simple airway manoeuvres, ventilation may not be possible due to airway abnormalities (e.g. facial trauma, epiglottitis, airway malformations).

If the obstruction is above the larynx (facial trauma, congenital facial abnormalities), supra-glottic airway devices (e.g. LMA) can be lifesaving. Nevertheless, expert help should be sought immediately as intubation may be needed using either conventional or optical laryngoscopy. Intubation by the non-expert would only be acceptable if no such expertise were available and it is not otherwise possible to oxygenate and ventilate a hypoxic child.

In the very rare situations when the clinician cannot ventilate the child and intubation is not possible, cricothyroidotomy should be considered.

Cricothyroidotomy

Needle cricothyroidotomy is a 'last resort' emergency technique indicated in cases of upper airway obstruction (e.g. laryngeal obstruction by oedema, foreign body or major facial trauma) and is a technique of default, i.e. only to be undertaken when ventilation by BMV or LMA and TT intubation have failed.

Cricothyroidotomy can be performed with a large-bore over-the-needle cannula. A syringe is connected to the cannula and gently aspirated as it punctures the cricothyroid membrane percutaneously, at an angle of 45° from the head. The trachea is situated just beneath the skin. Air aspiration confirms the correct position. The needle is removed and the cannula connected to a 3 or 3.5 mm TT adaptor and to a self-inflating bag system or directly via a 3-way tap, **with all ports open**, to an oxygen source. Oxygen is given by squeezing the bag (or obstructing the side port of the 3-way tap) for 1 second and 4 seconds are allowed for exhalation. Oxygen flow for this technique in l min^{-1} = age of the child in years (maximum 6 l min^{-1}).

Over-the-needle cannulae have high resistances. Small tidal volumes are delivered and there is no significant CO_2 removal. There is also a risk of barotraumas if the airway is completely obstructed above the cannula. The technique only provides temporary oxygenation until a definitive airway can be provided. Expert help must be sought as soon as possible.

Surgical tracheostomy should be reserved for skilled practitioners because it is a difficult technique with major risks, including haemorrhage, laryngeal tear, pneumomediastinum and subcutaneous emphysema.

Monitoring

Pulse oximetry

The clinical recognition of cyanosis may be difficult and is not reliable. Pulse oximetry enables continuous evaluation of the peripheral oxygen saturation of haemoglobin and is a valuable non-invasive method of monitoring the child. It provides an early indication of hypoxia and should be used during both stabilisation and transportation of the critically ill child. (Figure 4.20). A detecting probe is placed around a finger/toe (in the child) or hand/foot (in the infant). Ideally the pulse oximeter monitor should display a wave-form, a numerical percentage of oxygenation and produce a tone modulated sound. It is important to remember that it is a measure of oxygenation and does not indicate the adequacy of ventilation. Peripheral oxygen saturation readings should always be interpreted with reference to the inspired oxygen concentration. When peripheral perfusion is poor, recorded values will be unreliable. Furthermore in situations of cardiorespiratory arrest, circulatory failure or shock with severely reduced peripheral perfusion, pulse oximetry may be unrecordable.

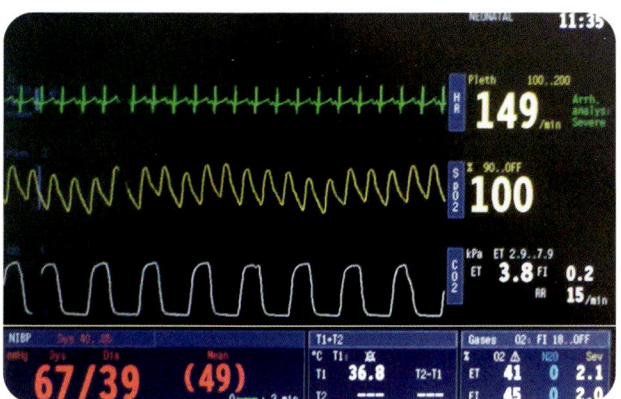

Figure 4.20 Pulse oximetry and capnography

End-tidal carbon dioxide monitoring (capnography)

Monitoring end-tidal CO_2 ($ETCO_2$) reliably confirms TT placement in a child weighing more than 2 kg with a perfusing rhythm. Its use is strongly recommended following intubation, and during the transportation of an intubated child. The CO_2 sampler should be placed as close to the TT as possible. The presence of a capnographic waveform for more than four ventilated breaths indicates that the TT is in the tracheobronchial tree, both in the presence of a perfusing rhythm and during cardiorespiratory arrest.

Continuous electronic capnography provides a waveform showing exhaled carbon dioxide during ventilation (Figure 4.20). Colourimetric detectors are also available and the presence of CO_2 is shown by changes in the colour of an indicator. Both types of devices are connected between the TT and the self-inflating bag.

The absence of exhaled CO_2 during cardiorespiratory arrest however, does not prove that the TT is misplaced, as pulmonary blood flow may be very low. If exhaled CO_2 is not detected during CPR, TT position should be confirmed using other methods, as described earlier. Exhaled CO_2 may also be reduced in low cardiac output states (especially in infants). Capnography may also provide information on the efficiency of chest compressions during CPR and a sudden rise in exhaled CO_2 can give an early indication of return of spontaneous circulation. Efforts should be made to improve chest compression quality if the exhaled carbon dioxide ($ETCO_2$) remains below 2 kPa as this may indicate low cardiac output and pulmonary blood flow.

False positives have been described with colourimetric dectors. If the detector is contaminated by acidic gastric contents or acidic drugs (e.g. adrenaline), the colour remains constant. False negatives occur when exhaled carbon dioxide is below the detection threshold, e.g. in asthma with severe bronchial obstruction.

Key learning points

▶ Airway management is the first priority in the care of the critically ill or injured child and is central to successful paediatric resuscitation

▶ The delivery of high-flow oxygen with the use of simple airway manoeuvres and BMV provides effective first-line management in the critically ill child

▶ Tracheal intubation is reserved for those experienced in the technique because it has many complications

Further reading

Blevin AE, McDouall SF, Rechner JA, Saunders TA, Barber VS, Young JD, Mason DG. A comparison of the laryngeal mask airway with the facemask and oropharyngeal airway for manual ventilation by first responders in children. Anaesthesia. 2009;64:1312-6.

Bhende MS, Thompson AE. Evaluation of an endtidal carbon dioxide detector during pediatric cardiopulmonary resuscitation. Pediatrics 1995; 95:395-399.

De Caen AR, Kleinman ME et al. Part 10: Pediatric basic and advanced life support 2010 International Consensus on Cardiopulmonary Rescucitation and Cardiovascular Care Science with Treatment Recommendations. Resuscitation 2010;81s:e213-259.

Ellis DY, et al. Cricoid pressure in emergency department rapid sequence tracheal intubations: a risk-benefit analysis. Ann Emerg Med 2007;50:653-65.

Gausche M, Lewis RJ, Stratton SJ, et al. Effect of out-of-hospital pediatric endotracheal intubation on survival and neurological outcome: a controlled clinical trial. JAMA 2000;283:783-90.

Eich C, Roessler M, Nemeth M, Russo SG, Heuer JF, Timmermann A. Characteristics and outcome of prehospital paediatric tracheal intubation attended by anaesthesia-trained emergency physicians. Resuscitation 2009;80:1371-7.

Ghai B, Wig J. Comparison of different techniques of laryngeal mask placement in children. Curr opin Anesth 2009; 22:4000-404.

Grein AJ, Weiner GM. Laryngeal mask airway versus bag-mask ventilation or endotracheal intubation for neonatal resuscitation. Cochrane Database Systemic Review 2005; CD003314.
http://www2.cochrane.org/reviews/en/ab003314.

Warner KJ, et al. Prehospital management of the difficult airway: a prospective cohort study. J Emerg Med 2009;36:257-65.

Weiss M, Dullenkopf A, Fischer JE, Keller C, Gerber AC European Paediatric Endotracheal Intubation Study Group. Prospective randomized controlled multi-centre trial of cuffed or uncuffed endotracheal tubes in small children. Br J Anaesth. 2009;103:867-73.

Zelicof-Paul A, Smith-Lockridge A, Schnadower D et al. Controversies in rapid sequence intubation in children. Current Opinion in Pediatrics 2005; 17: 355-362.

Rhythm Recognition

CHAPTER 5

Learning outcomes

To understand:
- ▶ The normal electrocardiogram (ECG) trace
- ▶ How to recognise cardiac rhythms associated with cardiorespiratory arrest
- ▶ The management of bradycardia
- ▶ The differentiation between sinus tachycardia (ST) and supraventricular tachycardia (SVT)
- ▶ The priorities of management in children with compensated and decompensated tachyarrhythmias

ECG monitoring

Once optimal ventilation and oxygenation have been established, all seriously ill children should have their ECG monitored as part of the assessment of their circulation. This facilitates the observation of heart rate changes, which are important indicators of the response to treatments, or the evolution of the disease process. It should be remembered that normal heart rates vary for physiological reasons (e.g. pain, pyrexia and wakefulness), and with age (Table 5.1).

Table 5.1: Heart rate ranges (beats min^{-1})

Age	Mean	Awake	Deep sleep
Newborn – 3 months	140	85 – 205	80 – 140
3 months – 2 years	130	100 – 180	75 – 160
2 – 10 years	80	60 – 140	60 – 90
> 10 years	75	60 – 100	50 – 90

Cardiac arrhythmias are more frequently the result, rather than the cause of acute illness in children. However, they do occasionally occur, particularly in children with:

- acquired cardiac disease (e.g. cardiomyopathy, myocarditis)
- congenital heart disease or following cardiac surgery
- electrolyte disturbances (e.g. renal disease)

Additionally, some medications (in therapeutic or toxic amounts) may also cause arrhythmias (e.g. digoxin, beta-blockers, tricyclic antidepressants).

By monitoring the ECG, it is possible to detect those arrhythmias that are (or have the potential to become) life-threatening.

Basic electrocardiography

The ECG trace represents electrical activity within the heart, and not the effectiveness of myocardial contraction or tissue perfusion. The child's clinical status needs to be considered alongside the ECG trace: **treat the patient not the monitor.**

When evaluating the ECG, possible artefacts may occur; detachment of ECG electrodes/leads can simulate asystole, whilst vibrations transmitted to the leads (e.g. during patient transportation) can mimic ventricular fibrillation (VF).

A normal ECG complex consists of a P wave, a QRS complex and a T wave (Figure 5.1).

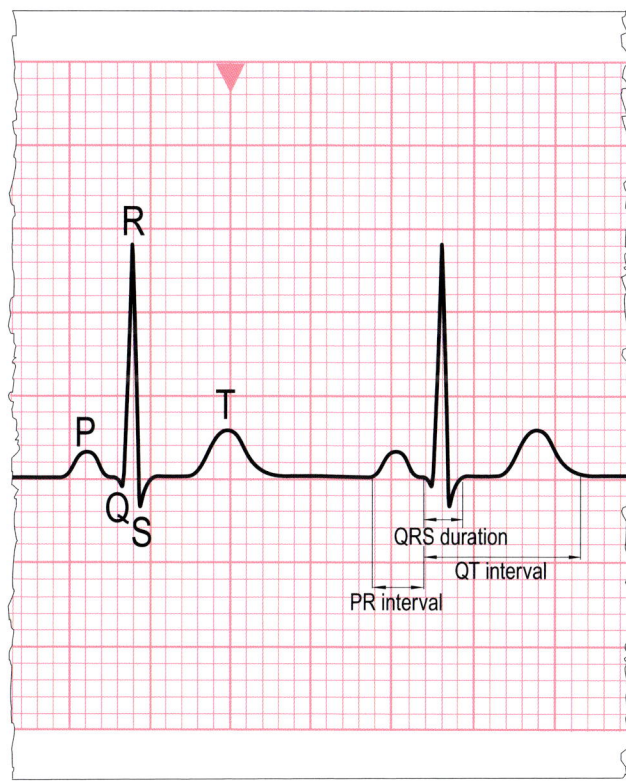

Figure 5.1 The normal ECG complex

The P wave represents electrical depolarisation of the atria. The time taken for depolarisation to pass through the atria, AV node and His-Purkinje system to the ventricles (Figure 5.2) is represented by the P-R interval. The QRS complex represents depolarisation of the ventricular myocardium. Ventricular repolarisation, in preparation for the next impulse, is represented by the ST segment and the

T wave. A prolonged QT interval is a risk factor for arrhythmias and sudden death.

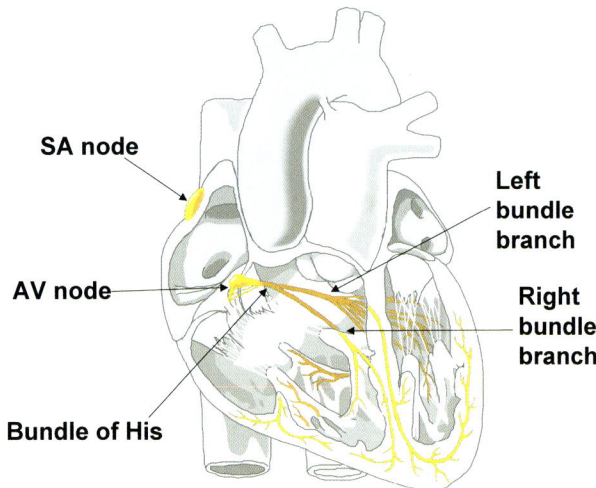

Figure 5.2 Electrical conduction through the heart

Cardiac rhythm disturbances

The approach to managing a child with a cardiac rhythm disturbance is summarised in Figure 5.3. This approach is based on determining the following 4 factors:

1. Presence or absence of circulation (i.e. a central pulse and other 'signs of life')

2. Clinical status – compensated (haemodynamically stable) or decompenstated (haemodynamically unstable)

3. Heart rate (bradycardia or tachycardia)

4. Width of QRS complexes on ECG (i.e. narrow or broad)

1. Presence of central pulse

Adopting the ABCDE approach, the rescuer must quickly establish the absence or presence of cardiac output, i.e. 'signs of life' and a palpable central pulse.

Absent pulse

The absence of 'signs of life' and no palpable central pulse indicates cardiorespiratory arrest. BLS should be started immediately. The rhythms associated with cardiorespiratory arrest are:

- asystole (or severe bradycardia)
- pulseless electrical activity (PEA)
- ventricular fibrillation (VF)
- pulseless ventricular tachycardia (VT)

The commonest cardiorespiratory arrest arrhythmia in paediatrics is asystole (generally preceded by progressive bradycardia). The term PEA describes the situation where there is organised electrical activity displayed on the ECG monitor but no cardiac output. The principles of managing both asystole and PEA are the provision of effective CPR, administration of adrenaline and the treatment of any underlying problems.

Both VF and pulseless VT are less common in children, but more likely in those with underlying cardiac disease. The priority of management in these arrhythmias is effective CPR and rapid defibrillation. VF and pulseless VT may also occur as a secondary rhythm during reperfusion of the myocardium during a cardiorespiratory arrest.

The management of cardiorespiratory arrest arrhythmias is outlined in Chapter 8.

Pulse present

If there is a central pulse present, the rescuer must determine whether or not the child is compensated (haemodynamically stable) or decompensated (haemodynamically unstable). (Chapter 2).

2. Clinical status

Compensated circulatory failure

The child with compensated circulatory failure, who is haemodynamically stable, must be monitored, including an ECG. If the ECG displays an arrhythmia, the child may need treatment, but it is reasonable to await expert help such as from a paediatric cardiologist. Preparations should be made to intervene (along the principles described below) should the child deteriorate and become decompensated.

Decompensated circulatory failure

The child who is decompensated (haemodynamically unstable) should be monitored and, if the ECG displays a life-threatening arrhythmia, the immediate interventions that may be required are outlined below. Urgent expert help must also be sought. This should include an anaesthetist or a paediatric intensivist as sedation or anaesthesia is required to manage a conscious child requiring cardioversion.

3. Heart rate

Both bradycardia and tachycardia are relatively common in paediatrics. Their defining heart rates are listed in Table 5.2.

Table 5.2: Bradycardia and tachycardia heart rates (beats min^{-1})		
Age	Bradycardia	Tachycardia
< 1 year	< 80	> 180
> 1 year	< 60	> 160

Bradycardia

Bradycardia may be due to hypoxia, acidosis and respiratory or circulatory failure, or it may be a pre-terminal event prior to cardiorespiratory arrest.

Managing the child with a cardiac arrhythmia

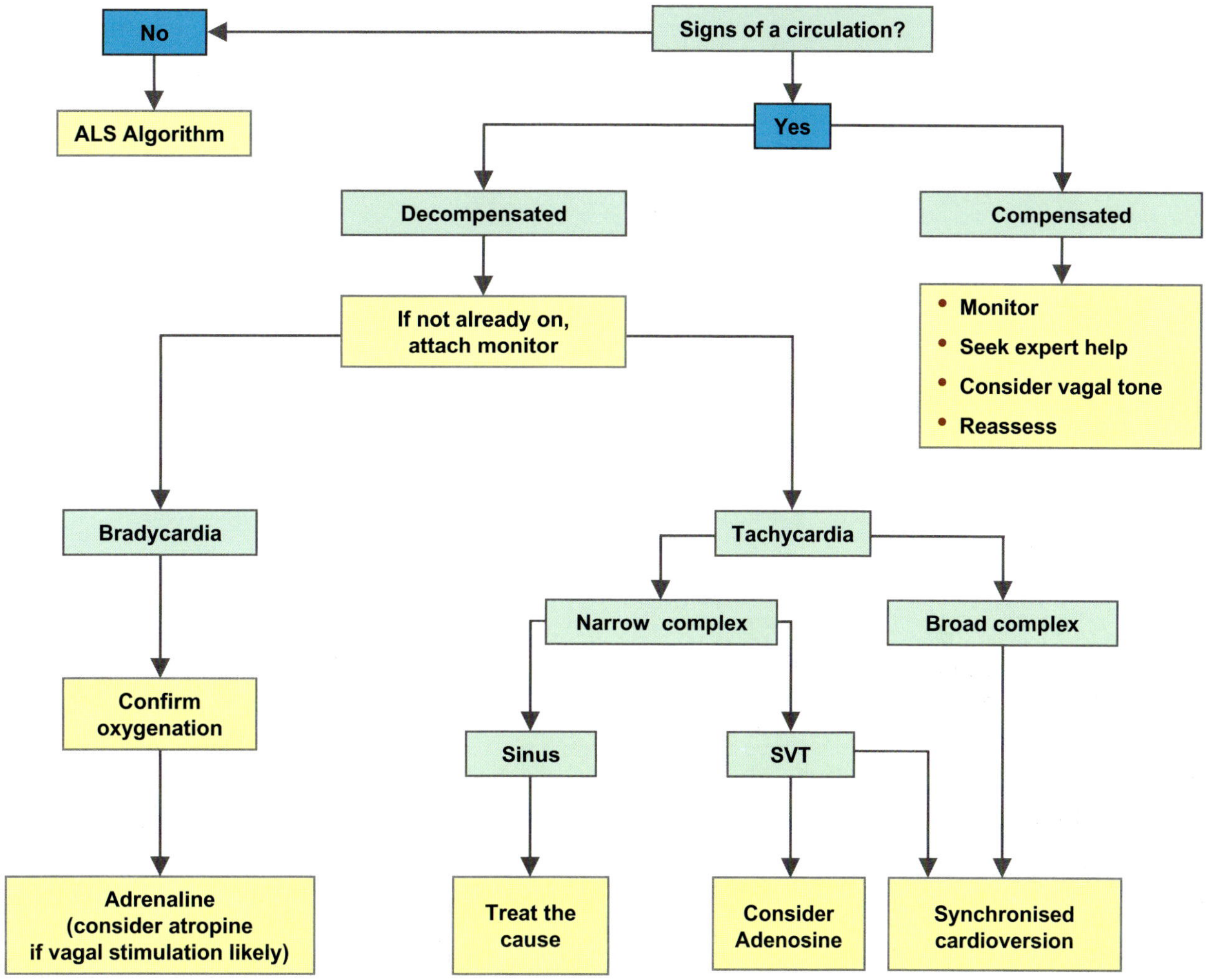

Figure 5.3 Approach to managing the child with an arrhythmia

A bradycardic child with signs of decompensation or a child with a rapidly dropping heart rate associated with poor systemic perfusion requires immediate oxygenation (airway opening, 100% oxygen administration and positive pressure ventilation as necessary). If the heart rate remains < 60 min^{-1} (all ages) and the child has decompensated circulatory failure, chest compressions must also be started. The cause of the bradycardia must be sought and treatment directed at the underlying cause.

By far the commonest causes of bradycardia in infants and children are hypoxia and vagal stimulation. Less commonly, hypothermia and hypoglycaemia can slow conduction through cardiac tissues and result in bradycardia. Infants and children with a history of heart surgery are at increased risk of sick sinus syndrome or heart block secondary to injury of the AV node or other parts of the conduction system.

Atropine is indicated when increased vagal tone is the cause of the bradycardia (e.g. induced by tracheal intubation or suctioning), Otherwise adrenaline is the medication of choice. Very occasionally, in a child with congenital heart disease, the bradycardia is due to complete heart block, and emergency cardiac pacing is required. Pacing is not indicated in children with bradycardia secondary to hypoxic/ischaemic myocardial insult or respiratory failure.

Tachycardia

An elevated heart rate is frequently the normal physiological response to anxiety, pain or pyrexia. This is sinus tachycardia (ST) and is managed by treating the primary cause.

Other causes of ST include:

- Respiratory conditions; early hypoxia, hypercarbia, obstructed airway and pneumothorax

- Circulatory conditions; hypovolaemia, cardiac failure, anaphylaxis or sepsis, pulmonary hypertension

- Miscellaneous causes; drugs, seizures.

The other cause of tachycardia is an arrhythmia, either supraventricular tachycardia (SVT) or ventricular tachycardia (VT). Of these, SVT is far more common in children. The priority of management is to establish whether or not the child is stable, or if they are displaying signs of

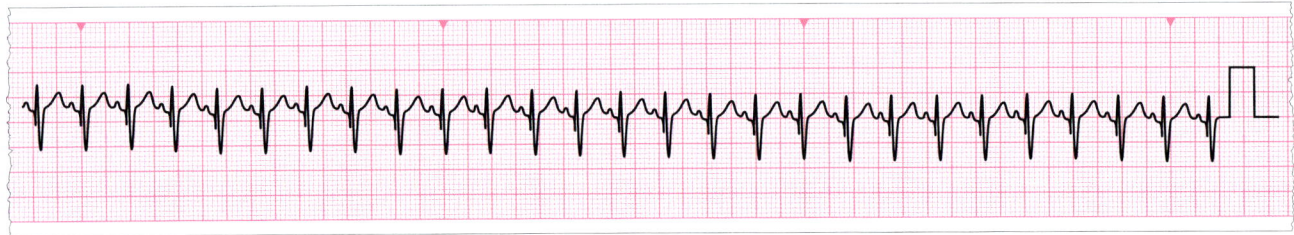

Figure 5.4 Sinus tachycardia rhythm strip

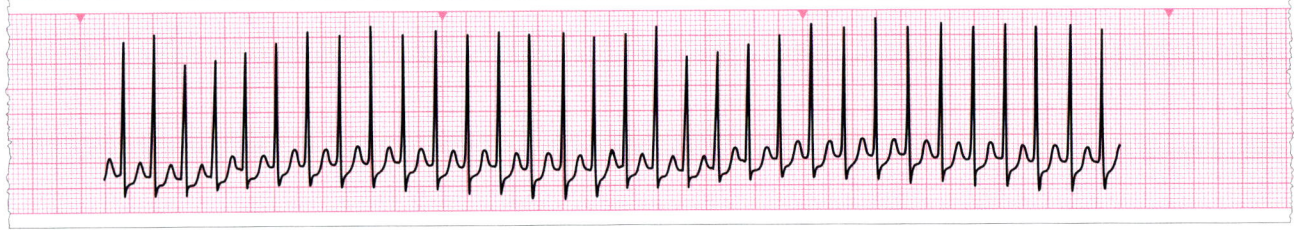

Figure 5.5 Supraventricular tachycardia rhythm strip

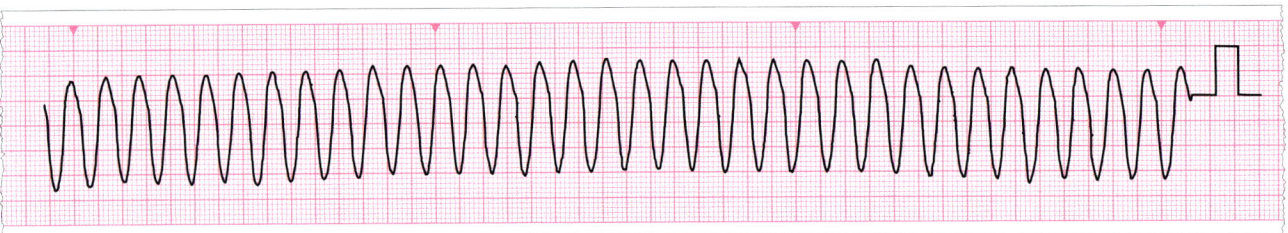

Figure 5.6 Ventricular tachycardia rhythm strip

circulatory decompensation. If the child is in a compensated state, expert help should be sought for definitive management.

The child who has decompensated circulatory failure requires chemical or electrical cardioversion whilst their ABCDE is continually assessed and appropriately supported.

4. Width of QRS complexes

In children with a tachycardia the most important thing to establish is whether this is ST or an abnormal rhythm (tachyarrhythmia). The history and clinical examination are key in determining this. The ECG features and width of the QRS complexes can also be helpful but it is always the child's clinical status that determines the urgency of management, regardless of the type of arrhythmia.

Narrow QRS complex tachycardia

Both ST (Figure 5.4) and SVT (Figure 5.5) have narrow QRS complexes, making it potentially difficult to differentiate between them. The clinical and ECG differences that help to make this distinction are listed in Table 5.3.

Broad QRS complex tachycardia

In children, broad complex tachycardia is uncommon; and usually due to an SVT. However, if uncertain, treat the rhythm as though it is VT as this has more immediately serious consequences if inadequately treated, i.e. it can deteriorate to VF or pulseless VT.

VT is usually found in a child who has underlying cardiac disease.

Ventricular tachycardia is a broad complex regular rhythm with P waves that are either absent or unrelated to the QRS complex (Figure 5.6). It can present with or without a pulse; pulseless VT is managed in the same manner as VF, i.e. it presents with cardiorespiratory arrest and needs CPR and urgent defibrillation.

The management of VT with a pulse involves urgent expert consultation, as it has the potential to rapidly deteriorate to pulseless VT or VF. The ongoing management of these children may involve cardioversion or amiodarone. An anaesthetist or paediatric intensivist should usually be present (in addition to a cardiologist if available) as amiodarone can cause hypotension and may result in rapid circulatory decompensation. If electrical cardioversion is required anaesthesia is necessary.

Supraventricular tachycardia

SVT is the most common primary cardiac arrhythmia observed in children. It is a paroxysmal, regular rhythm with narrow QRS complexes, caused by a re-entry mechanism through an accessory pathway or the atrioventricular conduction system. A heart rate of > 220 min^{-1} in infants or > 180 min^{-1} in children older than 1 year is highly suggestive of SVT. The other features that help to differentiate SVT from ST are listed in Table 5.3.

Table 5.3 Clinical and ECG differences between ST and SVT

	ST	SVT
History	Clues (e.g. pyrexia, fluid or blood loss)	Non specific Previous arrhythmia
Heart rate (beats min^{-1})	Infant < 220 Child < 180	Infant > 220 Child > 180
P wave	Present and normal (N.B. not clearly seen at heart rates > 200 min^{-1})	Absent or abnormal
Beat-to-beat variability (R – R)	Yes – can be altered with stimulation	None
Onset and end	Gradual	Abrupt

Management of SVT

Once a diagnosis of SVT is made, the child's clinical status will determine the management. As described previously, a child with compensated circulatory status should be referred for expert help. They may suggest that vagal manoeuvres be performed, as stimulation of the vagus nerve may slow atrioventricular conduction and result in a return to normal sinus rhythm.

Vagal manoeuvres

In infants and small children, this can be performed by soaking a flannel in ice cold water, and then placing it briefly over their face. In cooperative children, a Valsalva manoeuvre can be induced by asking the child to blow through a drinking straw. A variation on this is to blow through the outlet of a syringe in an effort to expel the plunger.

Adenosine

If intravascular access is already established in a conscious, compensated child with SVT, chemical cardioversion with adenosine may be possible. Adenosine should be given rapidly via a vein as close to the heart as possible, as it is metabolised by red blood cells as soon as it enters the bloodstream. A rapid bolus of 0.1 mg kg^{-1} should be followed with a flush of 2-5 ml 0.9% saline. If this dose is ineffective, it can be doubled (i.e. 0.2 mg kg^{-1}). The maximum dosages are 6 mg for the first attempt and 12 mg for the second. **Caution:** Adenosine can precipitate severe bronchospasm. It causes unpleasant feelings of impending doom in the child and should ideally only be given under the guidance of a paediatric cardiologist or intensivist. Adenosine should be used with caution in heart transplant recipients.

Cardioversion

The procedure for undertaking synchronised cardioversion is described in Chapter 7. It is the procedure of choice for decompensated children with SVT, particularly if they are unconscious. Cardioversion requires that anaesthesia or sedation must be arranged if the child is conscious. The first shock should be delivered at the energy level of 0.5 - 1 J kg^{-1}, and the second (if required) at 2 J kg^{-1}. If the SVT fails to convert after a second shock, amiodarone maybe recommended before further shocks are delivered. This should ideally be under the guidance of a paediatric cardiologist or paediatric intensivist.

Key learning points

- Life-threatening cardiac arrhythmias are more frequently the result, rather than the cause, of acute illness
- The child's clinical status dictates management priorities – *treat the patient not the monitor*
- The cause of the arrhythmia should be sought and treated

Further reading

Brierley J, Carcillo JA, Choong K et al. Clinical practice parameters for hemodynamic support of pediatric and neonatal septic shock: 2007 update from the American College of Critical Care Medicine. Crit Care Med 2009; 37:666-688.

Carcillo JA, Davis AL et al Role of early fluid resuscitation in pediatric septic shock. JAMA. 1991; 266:1242-1 245.

Carpenter TC, Stenmark KR. High-dose epinephrine is not superior to standard dose epinephrine in pediatric inhospital cardiopul monary arrest. Pediatrics. 1997; 99:403-408.

de Oliveira CF, de Oliveira DS, Gottschald AF, et al. ACCM/PALS haemodynamic support guidelines for paediatric septic shock: an outcomes comparison with and without monitoring central venous oxygen saturation. Intensive Care Med 2008; 34:1065-75.

Dauchot P, Gravenstein JS. Effects on atropine on the electrocardiogram in different age groups. Clin Pharmacol Ther 1971; 12:274-280.

Ditchey RV, Lindenfels JA. Potential adverse effects of volume loading on perfusion of vitals organs during closed-chest resuscitation. Circulation. 1984; 69:181-185.

Goetting MG, Paradis NA. High-dose of epinephrine improves outcome from pediatric cardiac arrest. Ann Emerg Med.1991; 20.22-26.

Graf W, Brutocao D et al. Admission glucose level as a predictor of survival and neurological outcome in pediatric submersion victims. Ann Neurol. 1991; 30:473-477.

Losek JD. Hypoglycaemia and the ABC's (sugar) of pediatric resuscitation. Ann Emerg Med 2000; 35:43-46.

Olasveengen TM, Sunde K, Brunborg C, Thowsen J, Steen PA, Wik L.Intravenous drug administration during out-of-hospital cardiac arrest: a randomized trial. J Am Med Assoc 2009;302:2222–9.

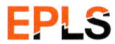

Michaud LJ, Rivara LP et al. Elevated initial blood glucose levels and poor outcome following severe brain injuries in children. J Trauma. 1991; 31:1356-1 362.

Patterson MD, Boenning DA, Klein BL et al. . the use of high-dose epinephrine for patients with out-of-hospital cardiopulmonary arrest refractory to prehospital interventions. Pediatr Emerg Care 2005;21:227-37.

Perondi MB, Reis AG, Paiva EF, Nadkarni VM, Berg RA. A comparison og high-dose and standard-dose epinephrine in children with cardiac arrest. N Eng J Med 2004;350:1722-30.

Srinivasan V, Spinella PC, Drott HR, Roth CL, Helfaer MA, Nadkarni V. Association of timing, duration and intensity of hyperglycemia with intensive care unit mortality in critically ill children. Pediatr Crit Care Med 2004;5:329-36.

Stiell IG, Wells GA, Field B, et al. Advanced cardiac life support in out-ofhospital cardiac arrest. N Engl J Med 2004;351:647–56.

Tenebein M. Continuous naloxone infusion for opiate poisoning in infancy. J Pediatr. 1988; 105:645-648, 1988.

Emergency Circulatory Access, Fluid Administration and Medications

CHAPTER 6

Learning outcomes

To understand:

▸ The requirement for circulatory access during resuscitation

▸ The different routes of emergency circulatory access and their appropriate use

▸ The advantages and potential complications of intraosseous access

▸ Central venous access

▸ The type and volume of fluids to be administered in the emergency situation

▸ The indications, dosages and actions of the first-line medications used in cardiorespiratory arrest

Circulatory access

Once the airway is patent and adequate ventilation of the child is established, the rescuers need to focus on the circulation.

Access to the circulation is important for all critically ill children, but during cardiorespiratory arrest it is essential that it is achieved rapidly for the following reasons:

- administration of medications (e.g. adrenaline)
- administration of fluids
- obtaining blood samples

Chest compressions, if required, should not be interrupted, except to perform defibrillation.

If there is an intravenous (IV) cannula already in situ, its patency must be confirmed before use. Any medications must be followed with a bolus 'flush' of 2-5 ml 0.9% saline.

The intraosseous and intravenous routes are strongly preferred to the tracheal route. Until either intravenous or intraosseous access is secured however, the tracheal route may be used for the administration of lipid-soluble medications such as adrenaline, atropine and naloxone. The pharmacokinetic effect on drugs given via the tracheal route is highly variable, making it an undesirable route. The optimal drug dosages via the tracheal route are unknown owing to the variability in alveolar drug absorption. Although atropine, adrenaline, naloxone, lidocaine and vasopressin are absorbed from the tracheobronchial tree, much lower blood concentrations result than if the same dose were given intravascularly.

Catecholamines should ideally be infused through a dedicated line; continuous catecholamine therapy may be required as part of the ongoing resuscitation of the child.

The use of scalp veins during resuscitation is not advisable owing to the risk of extravasation leading to potential tissue necrosis. Their use may also interfere with the management of the airway and ventilation.

The largest possible IV cannula should be sited in peripheral veins such as in the antecubital fossa, the long saphenous vein, the back of the hand (or feet in smaller children) should be sited or the intraosseous (IO) route secured as soon as possible.

There is good quality evidence in both adult and paediatric studies to show that IO access is safe and effective, therefore this route is therefore far preferable to tracheal administration. The tracheal route should be used only if there is no alternative. Semi-automated devices for inserting IO needles are available. Although there are few data to support their use in children during CPR, reports of their use in other circumstances have shown them to be effective.

Intraosseous access

In cardiorespiratory arrest, the IO route is the emergency circulatory access route of choice. Placement of an IO cannula involves insertion of a needle through the skin, periosteum and cortex of a bone, into the medullary cavity. The IO route should be **the first choice** in any situation where the child's clinical status is severely compromised (i.e. they are in a decompensated state) or they have suffered a cardiorespiratory arrest. The main advantages of IO access are:

- The relative ease and speed of insertion

- It can be used to deliver all resuscitation fluids, medications and blood-derived products

- It allows rapid adequate plasma concentration of medications similar to that of central venous administration (more rapid and reliable than that achieved through a peripheral IV)

- It permits bone marrow aspiration, which can be used for analysis. In this situation, the laboratory should be informed as the fat in a marrow sample may cause damage to auto-analysers.

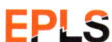

Chapter 6 Emergency Circulatory Access, Fluid Administration and Medications

Insertion of an intraosseous cannula

Before undertaking this procedure, the appropriate equipment must be available and there should be no contraindications to IO insertion.

Insertion site – anatomical landmarks

The usual site for insertion of an IO cannula is 2-3 cm below the tuberosity on the anteromedial surface of the tibia. Other sites that can be used include the lower end of the tibia (approximately 3 cm above the medial malleolus) or on the lateral aspect of the distal femur (approximately 3 cm above the lateral condyle). These sites specifically avoid the growth plates of the bones (Figure 6.1).

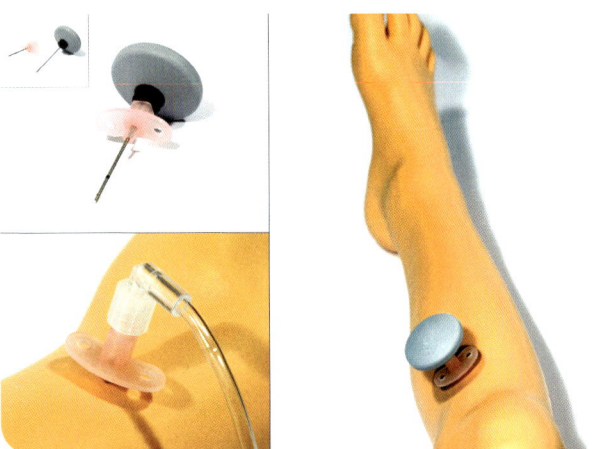

Figure 6.2 Intraosseous cannula and trocar

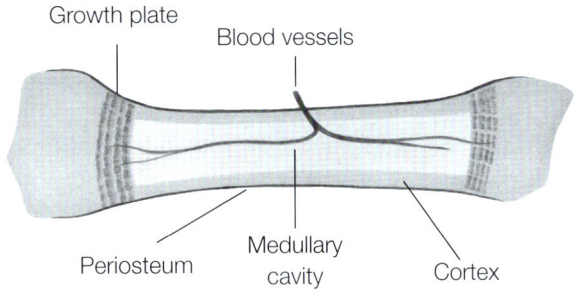

Figure 6.1 Anatomy of a long bone

Contraindications

Contraindications to the insertion of an IO include osteogenesis imperfecta ('brittle bone' disease) and haemophilia or other known coagulopathies. Intraosseous cannulation should not be through an area of infected skin or wounds. Fractured bones must not be used, nor should the cannula be inserted into a bone immediately distal to a fracture site, as this may predispose to the development of compartment syndrome.

Equipment required

1. IO cannulae

There are several designs of manually inserted intraosseous cannulae available commercially, but they are generally either of a 'screw' type design or needles with a hole at the tip, and on either side of the end of the cannula (Figure 6.2).

Intraosseous cannulae have a trocar and come in a variety of sizes. Generally, it is recommended that size 18 gauge is used for a newborn-6 months of age, 16 gauge for a child between 6-18 months, and 14 gauge for children > 18 months.

There are also a number of intraosseous 'guns' or drills available (Figure 6.3). These are loaded with the cannula and then activated to 'fire' or drill a cannula in to the medullary cavity; they require specialist training prior to use.

If there is no dedicated IO cannula available, bone marrow aspiration or spinal (lumbar puncture) needles can be used.

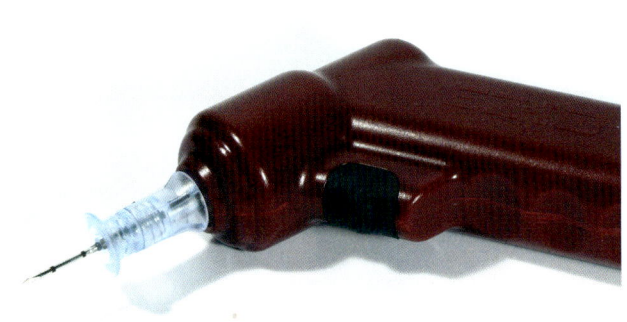

Figure 6.3 EZ IO complete

Additional IO cannulae should be available in case of insertion difficulties or the need to secure further vascular access (e.g. infusion of vasoactive medications; in cases of trauma where large volumes of fluid require to be rapidly infused).

2. Alcohol-based skin preparation solution

This minimises the risk of infection.

3. Three-way tap with integrated IV extension tubing

This is primed with 0.9% saline and attached to a syringe also filled with 0.9% saline (to minimise the risk of air emboli, confirm correct placement and allow for flushing of medications).

4. Syringe

This is to aspirate bone marrow once the IO is inserted (to obtain sample and/or confirm correct position).

5. Emergency medications and/or fluids

Have these to hand to ensure prompt delivery when access is achieved.

6. Local anaesthetic agent

If the child is still conscious, this should be considered to minimise pain, along the intended track of the IO cannula.

EUROPEAN PAEDIATRIC LIFE SUPPORT

Technique for manual insertion of an IO cannula

1. Identify the site to be accessed

2. Clean the skin around selected site with an alcohol-based solution

3. Infiltrate the skin through to the periosteum with local anaesthetic agent (i.e. 1% lidocaine) if appropriate

4. Immobilise the limb with non-dominant hand (ensure no hands are placed under the limb)

5. Using the dominant hand, the rescuer should grasp the needle and position it at a 90% angle on the skin at the prepared site

6. Using a firm rotating action, the needle should be advanced (approximately 1-2 cm) until loss of resistance is felt; this 'give' indicates penetration of the cortex

7. Unscrew and withdraw the trocar

8. The 3-way tap with integrated IV extension tubing should be attached and marrow aspirated and/or fluid flushed in to the cannula to confirm position. If it is vital to obtain a marrow sample this can be attempted at this point. However, this must not delay administration of adrenaline in cardiorespiratory arrest.

9. Administer resuscitation medications and/or fluid boluses as indicated (Figure 6.4). It should be noted that, with the smaller size cannulae, a fluid bolus may be easier to deliver with a 20 ml rather than a 50 ml syringe

10. Although the cannula will be stable once correctly sited, it is advisable to secure it further to prevent accidental dislodgement, particularly during transfer of the child to a definitive care facility

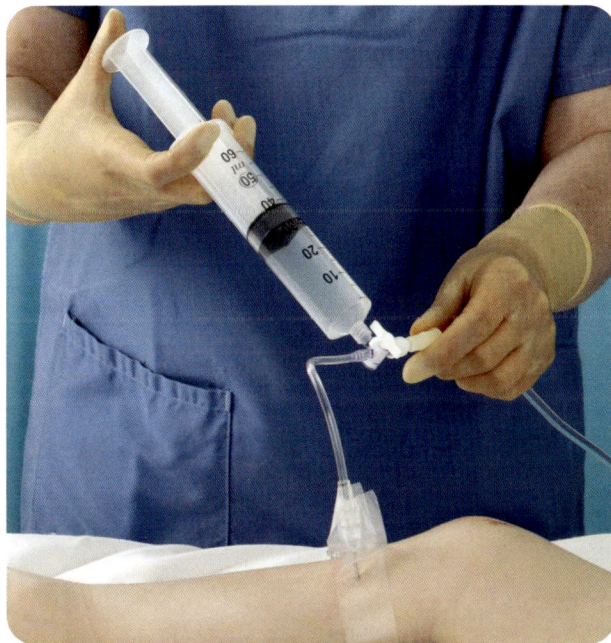

Figure 6.4 Administration of fluid via a secured intraosseous cannula

Potential complications

Although these are uncommon, complications can occur. These include:

- Extravasation
  True extravasation ('tissuing') of an IO cannula is uncommon. However, transient trivial swelling of subcutaneous tissue is commonly seen as fluid leaks from the marrow cavity into surrounding tissues. If the swelling does not rapidly subside or there is concern that the cannula is misplaced, the rescuer should withdraw a small amount of fluid; this aspirate should be blood stained if the cannula is in the correct place.

- Embolism
  There is a small risk (estimated at < 1%) of fat or bone marrow embolism

- Infection
  (e.g. osteomyelitis or cellulitis)

- Compartment syndrome

- Skin necrosis

- Fracture

The potential for any of the listed complications other than fracture can be minimised by removing the cannula as soon as alternative secure intravenous access has been obtained.

Central venous access

Continuous infusions of inotropes, corrosive agents (e.g. potassium) and the monitoring of central venous pressure are best performed by the central venous route. It also permits rapid infusion of large volumes of fluid. There is a quicker onset of action and an earlier peak level of resuscitation drugs, if they are given via this route. Vasospasm and extravasation are less likely to occur with central venous than with peripheral access. However, insertion of a central venous line in a child requires practice and can be time consuming.

Urgent insertion of central venous line

The following equipment is needed:

- Alcohol-based solution

- Lidocaine 1% for local anaesthesia with a 2 ml syringe and G23 needle (in the conscious child, consider a general anaesthetic)

- Syringe of 0.9% saline

- Suture material

- Infusion set

- Adhesive tape

- Over-the-needle cannula

A G20 or larger needle should be used for rapid volume expansion and the administration of drugs. This can also be used to place a central line using a Seldinger technique.

Complications

General complications include haematoma, venous obstruction, thrombosis, thrombophlebitis, air embolism and sepsis.

Specific complications of superior vena caval access (i.e. via the subclavian or internal jugular vein) include haemothorax, pneumothorax, cardiac tamponade, arrhythmias, diaphragmatic paralysis, Horner's syndrome and puncture of the internal carotid artery.

Those seen in securing inferior vena caval access (i.e. via the femoral vein) include intestinal perforation, haematoma of the inguinal or retroperitoneal areas, septic arthritis of the hip and renal vein thrombosis.

Femoral vein

The inguinal site is most commonly used during cardiopulmonary resuscitation as its distance from the head and chest allows cannulation without interrupting the management of the airway and breathing. This is a technique best carried out by the experienced clinician.

Technique

1. Place the leg in slight external rotation.

2. Clean the skin at the site of insertion.

3. Identify the puncture site. The vein is directly medial to the femoral artery. If the artery is not palpable, its location corresponds to the point midway between the anterior superior iliac spine and the pubic symphysis. During chest compressions, pulsations can be felt in the femoral artery and vein.

4. If the child is aware of pain, lidocaine 1% should be used to infiltrate the puncture site. General anaesthesia should be considered in the conscious child.

5. Attach the cannula with a needle to a saline-filled syringe, introduce it at a 45° angle, pointing the bevel of the needle towards the child's head, directly over the vein and keep the syringe in line with the child's thigh.

6. Advance the needle, pulling back on the plunger once the needle is below the surface of the skin.

7. As soon as blood flows back into the syringe, stop advancing it.

8. Gently remove the needle with the syringe, leaving the cannula in the vein.

9. Occlude the end of the cannula to prevent blood loss.

10. Confirm the location of the cannula by attempting to aspirate blood and if blood is obtained, flush the cannula with 0.9% saline and attach it to a pre-flushed 3-way tap.

11. Secure the cannula.

Fluid administration for volume resuscitation

Intravascular fluids are primarily administered to restore circulatory volume and ensure adequate perfusion of vital organs.

During cardiorespiratory arrest, hypovolaemia is often a primary contributory factor and fluid resuscitation may play a critical part in achieving return of spontaneous circulation.

The administration of fluids is also indicated for any child exhibiting signs of circulatory failure (e.g. decreased skin perfusion, prolonged capillary refill time, hypotension). The only children in whom caution is advised are those in suspected cardiogenic shock where the heart is unable to deal with the volume load or those with diabetic ketoacidosis.

Fluid volumes

During the resuscitation of a child with compromised circulation due to hypovolaemia (including sepsis and anaphylaxis), initial resuscitation fluid is administered as a bolus of 20 ml kg^{-1}. The child's circulatory status should then be reassessed and if signs of circulatory failure persist, this should be repeated. Signs of over-transfusion are moist sounds ('crackles') at the lung bases and jugular venous distension in children or liver distension in infants.

If circulatory failure is due to other causes, such as cardiac failure, a smaller initial volume (10 ml kg^{-1}) should be used. The effect of each smaller bolus should be carefully assessed to ensure that fluid administration is not causing worsening of the circulation (e.g. crackles at the lung bases and size of liver edge).

If there is no improvement in circulatory status following 40-60 ml kg^{-1}, ongoing losses must be suspected (e.g. diarrhoeal fluid, bleeding). In cases of trauma, a surgical referral should be made for full patient evaluation as haemostasis may only be achieved by surgery.

In septic shock, fluid resuscitation is specifically required as vasodilatation may be considerable and there may be a relatively hypovolaemic state. Up to 60-80 ml kg^{-1} of volume expansion is often required in the first hour of resuscitation; larger volumes (100-200 ml kg^{-1}) can be required within the first few hours. Inotropes (and intubation) may also be required in children with septic shock and considered at an early stage e.g. after 40 ml kg^{-1}.

Fluids must be infused during cardiorespiratory arrest if hypovolaemic shock is a likely cause of the arrest. However, excessive amounts of fluid may be harmful in these circumstances and in post-resuscitation states. Measurement of BP is of little help in determining circulatory status as it remains normal in compensated circulatory failure and only starts to drop as decompensation develops.

The aim in the management of hypovolaemic shock is to prevent the onset of decompensated circulatory failure, as this may lead to irreversible cardiorespiratory failure and death.

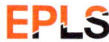

The principles of management adhere to ABCDE (airway, breathing, circulation, disability, exposure) with fluid administration forming part of the 'C' phase of resuscitation.

Types of fluid

In the initial phase of resuscitation, isotonic salt solutions should be used. There are no clear advantages between using crystalloid or colloid solutions. Glucose containing solutions (such as dextrose saline) should never be used for volume replacement as they can cause hyponatraemia and hyperglycaemia, which in turn, can lead to further fluid loss.

Crystalloids

Examples of appropriate resuscitation crystalloids include:

- 0.9% saline
- Ringer's lactate
- Hartmann's solution

Crystalloids are cheap, readily available and do not cause allergic reactions. They are however, less efficient than colloids at increasing circulating volume within the intravascular space, as they rapidly move into the surrounding interstitium; only 50-75% of the administered volume remains in the intravascular compartment. Therefore, to correct the initial circulatory deficit volume, 1.5-2 times this volume has to be infused; this may be poorly tolerated in children with underlying cardiac or respiratory disease, and pulmonary oedema may occur.

Crystalloids are indicated to replace fluid loss from the interstitial space and to correct electrolyte deficiencies, as seen in patients with burns or who are dehydrated.

Large quantities of saline, but not Ringer's lactate, may induce hyperchloraemic acidosis, therefore monitoring of the blood electrolyte concentrations should occur.

Infusion of fluids containing potassium must be avoided, particularly in children with anuria or oliguria, as hyperkalaemia could arise.

Glucose solutions should never be used for volume expansion as they can cause hyperglycaemia, resulting in osmotic diuresis. This increases urine production and so increases circulatory volume loss. Glucose solutions should only be used to correct hypoglycaemia following measurement of blood sugar levels: 2 ml kg^{-1} of 10% glucose is given and the patient's blood sugar should be re-measured shortly afterwards to ensure it is within the normal range. In the newborn 2.5 ml kg^{-1} of 10% glucose may be given initially to correct hypoglycaemia.

Colloids

Examples of colloids include:

- Human albumin (4.5%) solution
- Fresh frozen plasma (FFP)
- Gelatin solutions (e.g. Gelofusin)
- Starch solutions

Colloids are relatively expensive and less readily available than crystalloids. Colloids should be not be used in anaphylaxis because of the potential risk of allergic reaction. The main reason for considering the use of colloids in resuscitation is that they remain in the vascular space for longer, and may therefore increase the circulatory volume more efficiently than crystalloids. The use of human albumin solution (HAS) has been advocated for the ongoing management of sepsis.

Blood products

The administration of blood products is reserved for situations where there is a specific indication for their use (i.e. blood loss or coagulopathy). If the infusion of 40 ml kg^{-1} (i.e. 20 ml kg^{-1} bolus x 2) does not improve the circulatory status of a child who has suffered trauma, transfusion of blood must be considered, as well as urgent surgical referral.

In an emergency, Group O Rhesus-negative 'flying squad' blood or type specific uncross-matched blood may be used for transfusion until fully cross-matched blood is available.

Fresh frozen plasma should only be used in resuscitation situations for the treatment of specific coagulation abnormalities.

The risks of blood product administration must always be borne in mind.

First-line resuscitation medications

Only a few medications are indicated during the initial resuscitation phase of a child in cardiorespiratory arrest. Administration of medications should be considered only after adequate ventilation and chest compressions have been established, and in the case of a shockable arrhythmia (VF or pulseless VT), following delivery of the first three defibrillation shocks.

For safety reasons, as well as speed and ease of use, the use of pre-filled medication syringes is advocated.

All medications administered should be followed by a flush of 2-5 ml 0.9% saline to ensure they reach the circulation and to minimise the risks of interactions with any other medications or fluids administered via the same cannula. All medications and fluids should be recorded as they are administered and then documented at the end of the resuscitation attempt.

Adrenaline

Indication for use:

- cardiorespiratory arrest of any aetiology
- bradycardia < 60 min^{-1} with decompensated circulatory shock after the initial steps to restore satisfactory oxygenation and ventilation have been taken

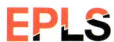

- hypotension with anaphylaxis

It should be given as soon as circulatory access has been achieved in non-shockable rhythms and after **the 3rd defibrillation in shockable ones.**

Dosage: in cardiorespiratory arrest or bradycardia with decompensated circulatory failure 10 mcg kg^{-1} (or 0.1 ml kg^{-1} of 1:10 000 solution). This is repeated every 3-5 minutes as necessary.

Actions: adrenaline is an endogenous, directly acting sympathomimetic amine with both alpha and beta adrenergic activity. In the dose used in resuscitation, adrenaline produces vasoconstriction, which results in increased cerebral and coronary perfusion pressure. It also increases myocardial contractility and may facilitate defibrillation success.

Alpha adrenergic effects cause splanchnic and mucocutaneous vasoconstriction with increased systolic and diastolic blood pressure. Beta-1 and 2 adrenergic effects increase the force and rate of myocardial contractions, and cause vascular smooth muscle vasodilatation and bronchiolar smooth muscle relaxation. Adrenaline's pharmacological effects are dose-related.

In cardiorespiratory arrest, alpha adrenergic- mediated vasoconstriction is the most important pharmacological action of adrenaline as this increases the diastolic pressure, so enhancing coronary perfusion and oxygen delivery to the heart. This is a critical determinant for successful resuscitation.

Other beneficial effects include:

- Elevation of systolic BP
- Increased tendency for a normal cardiac perfusing rhythm to develop during cardiorespiratory resuscitation
- Enhanced contractile state of the heart and stimulated spontaneous cardiac contractions
- Increased amplitude of ventricular fibrillation
- Increased intensity of ventricular fibrillation, so increasing the likelihood of successful response to defibrillation (i.e. return to normal rhythm)

The most commonly observed rhythms in the paediatric patient with cardiorespiratory arrest are asystole and bradyarrhythmia; adrenaline may generate a perfusing rhythm in these children. As the action of catecholamines may be depressed by acidosis careful attention to oxygenation, ventilation and circulation is essential (i.e. ABCDE).

Catecholamines are inactivated by alkaline solutions and should never be given simultaneously with sodium bicarbonate via the same vascular access cannula. If both these medications are to be used, their administration must be separated by a bolus of 0.9% saline (2-5 ml) if only one cannula is available.

If circulatory access is not present, and cannot be quickly obtained, but the patient has a tracheal tube in place, consider giving adrenaline 100 mcg kg^{-1} via the tracheal tube. This is the least satisfactory route (see routes of drug administration above).

Asystole, pulseless electrical activity (PEA), ventricular fibrillation (VF) and pulseless ventricular tachycardia (VT) all require the same dosage regime, 10 mcg kg^{-1} of adrenaline (or 0.1 ml kg^{-1} of a 1: 10 000 solution [1 mg 10 ml^{-1}]) by intravenous or intraosseous route. Adrenaline is given every 3-5 minutes (or every two loops of 2 minutes of CPR), starting after the 3rd defibrillation for the shockable rhythm protocol.

In newborns, the maximum dose is 10-30 mcg kg^{-1} (or 0.1- 0.3 ml kg^{-1} of a 1:10 000 solution) by the intravenous or intraosseous route. The tracheal route is not recommended, but if it is used, higher doses (50-100 mcg kg^{-1}) of adrenaline may be needed. Large doses of adrenaline may increase the risk of intracranial haemorrhage in newborns, especially in preterm infants.

The half-life of adrenaline is short (2 minutes) and doses are repeated until the desired effect is achieved; hence, a continuous infusion of adrenaline may occasionally be helpful once spontaneous circulation is restored.

The haemodynamic effects are dose-related:

- Low-dose infusions (< 0.1 mcg kg^{-1} min^{-1}) produce beta-adrenergic effects
- High-dose infusions (> 0.1 mcg kg^{-1} min^{-1}) produce alpha-adrenergic mediated vasoconstriction

Precaution: boluses of adrenaline should be administered via a secure vascular (IV or IO) cannula. If ongoing post-resuscitation care requires an adrenaline infusion, this should be through a central venous cannula as extravasation can cause severe tissue injury.

Adrenaline frequently causes tachycardia and may produce or exacerbate ventricular ectopics.

Higher doses of adrenaline (100 mcg kg^{-1}) administered by the vascular route are not recommended routinely as they do not improve survival or neurological outcome after cardiorespiratory arrest.

They may be required in exceptional circumstances (e.g. adrenoceptor blocker overdose). High-dose infusion regimens may produce excessive vasoconstriction, compromising blood flow in the extremities, mesentery of the bowel and the kidneys. Adrenaline causes tachycardia and may produce or exacerbate ventricular ectopics.

Amiodarone

Indication for use: refractory ventricular fibrillation or pulseless VT. If VF or pulseless VT persists after the 3rd defibrillation shock, a dose of amiodarone should be given with adrenaline. This can be repeated after the 5th shock if defibrillation is still unsuccessful.

Dosage: 5 mg kg^{-1}.

Actions: amiodarone is a membrane-stabilising anti-arrhythmic medication that increases the duration of the action potential and refractory period in both atrial and ventricular myocardium. Atrioventricular conduction is also slowed, and a similar effect is seen in accessory pathways. Amiodarone has a mild negative inotropic action and causes peripheral vasodilatation through non-competitive alpha-blocking effects. The hypotension that occurs with IV amiodarone is related to the rate of delivery and is due more to the solvent (Polysorbate 80 and benzyl alcohol), which causes histamine release, than the drug itself. The oral form is not well absorbed but the intravenous form has been successfully used for tachyarrhythmia management.

Precaution: amiodarone should be given as a pre-filled syringe preparation or diluted in 5% glucose. Ideally, it should be administered via a central vascular (IV or IO) route as it can cause thrombophlebitis. If it has to be given peripherally it should be liberally flushed with 0.9% saline or 5% glucose.

In the treatment of shockable rhythms, give an initial IV bolus dose of amiodarone 5 mg kg^{-1} after the third shock. Repeat the dose after the fifth shock if still in VF/VT.

If defibrillation was successful but VF/VT recurs, amiodarone can be repeated (unless two doses have already been injected) and a continuous infusion started.

In supraventricular tachycardia (SVT), amiodarone must be injected slowly (over 20-60 minutes) to avoid hypotension. Systemic BP and ECG should be continuously monitored.

Other rare but significant adverse effects are bradycardia and polymorphic ventricular tachycardia.

Glucose

Indication for use: documented hypoglycaemia. Neonatal, child and adult data show that both hyper- and hypo-glycaemia are associated with worsened outcome after cardiorespiratory arrest. Plasma glucose concentrations should be monitored closely in any ill or injured child, including after cardiorespiratory arrest. Do not give glucose-containing fluids during CPR except for the treatment of hypoglycaemia. Hyper- and hypo- glycaemia should be avoided following ROSC but tight glucose control has not shown survival benefits when compared with moderate glucose control in adults and increased the risk of hypoglycaemia in neonates, children and adults.

Infants have high glucose requirements and low glycogen storage. They can readily become hypoglycaemic during coma, circulatory and respiratory failure. It is therefore necessary to monitor closely their blood glucose concentrations.

The clinical signs of hypoglycaemia and shock may have similarities, i.e. hypotension, tachycardia, decreased peripheral perfusion and sweating.

Dosage: 200 mg kg^{-1} (or 2 ml kg^{-1}) of 10% glucose solution. Newborn 2.5 ml kg^{-1} of 10% glucose solution

Re-checking the blood glucose value should be performed shortly afterwards, e.g. 2 minutes following administration to determine if further dosages are required.

Actions: glucose is a principal energy substrate of all body tissues including the brain and myocardial cells. Low blood levels mean that myocardial contractility and therefore cardiac output, may be reduced.

Precaution: the association between hypoglycaemia and seizures is well documented. Prevention of seizures is essential to minimise the risk of neurological insult. Additionally, studies have shown a correlation between poor neurological outcome and hyperglycaemia. It is therefore important that blood glucose measurement is repeated regularly to ensure it is maintained within the normal range.

Once resuscitation has been completed, a continuous infusion of a glucose-containing solution is preferable to serial bolus therapy with hypertonic glucose. Repeated hyperglycaemia may increase serum osmolarity with the risk of osmotic diuresis. There is also a risk of intraventricular haemorrhage in the premature neonate if bolus(es) of hypertonic solutions is/are used. A risk of cutaneous necrosis exists if hypertonic glucose leaks into surrounding tissues.

Sodium bicarbonate

This is not a first-line resuscitation medication. Studies have shown that the routine use of sodium bicarbonate does not improve outcome.

Indication for use: The routine use of sodium bicarbonate is not recommended. It may be considered in prolonged arrest and it has a specific role in management of hyperkalaemia and the arrhythmias associated with tricyclic antidepressant.

Dosage: the initial dose is 1 mmol kg^{-1}. This equates to 1 ml kg^{-1} of 8.4% solution, although in newborns and infants < 3 months the weaker concentration (i.e. 4.2%) solution should be used to limit the osmotic load.

The decision to give further doses should be based on blood gas analysis.

Actions: sodium bicarbonate is administered to reverse metabolic acidosis. However, as it elevates PaCO$_2$ levels, the administration of sodium bicarbonate may worsen existing respiratory acidosis, a possible cause of the cardiorespiratory arrest. It may also cause paradoxical intracellular acidosis, thus worsening cellular function (e.g. myocardial dysfunction may be induced by the acidosis within myocardial cells). Some of the specific effects of sodium bicarbonate administration include:

- carbon dioxide production which diffuses into cells and exacerbates the intracellular acidosis
- left displacement of the oxyhaemoglobin dissociation curve inhibiting oxygen release to the tissues
- intracellular shift of potassium
- hypernatraemia due to the high, osmotically active, sodium content
- lowered VF threshold
- decreased plasma calcium

The potential negative effects of sodium bicarbonate outweigh any benefits unless the metabolic acidosis is severe, and even then it should be used with caution.

Precautions: arterial blood gas analysis does not reflect venous or tissue pH and should be interpreted with caution. Care should also be taken to ensure that an adequate flush of 0.9% saline is given between delivery of sodium bicarbonate and any other medications via the same cannula, as incompatibilities may occur.

Atropine

Indication for use: Bradycardia resulting from vagal stimulation. There is no evidence that atropine has any benefit in asphyxial bradycardia or asystole and its routine use has been removed from the advanced life support algorithms.

Dosage: 20 mcg kg^{-1}.

This dose may be repeated but, once the vagus nerve has been fully blocked, there is no further beneficial effect; the minimum dose is 100 mcg.

Actions: Atropine blocks the effect of the vagus nerve on the sinoatrial (SA) and atrioventricular (AV) nodes, increasing sinus automaticity, facilitating AV node conduction and increasing heart rate. The functions of the vagus nerve include pupillary constriction, contraction of the gut and production of salivary and gastro-intestinal secretions. During resuscitation, atropine may be of benefit in treating bradycardia which accompanies actions that result in vagal stimulation such as laryngoscopy.

Precautions: there is a potential paradoxical effect (i.e. further bradycardia) if a very small dose is used. A minimum dose of 100 mcg is therefore recommended.

Calcium

Calcium is essential to myocardial contraction. Its routine administration does not improve the outcome of cardiorespiratory arrest, but high plasma concentrations achieved after injection may be harmful to the ischaemic myocardium and may also impair cerebral recovery. The administration of calcium during cardiorespiratory arrest has been associated with increased mortality.

Indication for use: Routine administration of calcium in advanced life support is not recommended. It is only indicated for the treatment of documented hypocalcaemia, hyperkalaemia, hypermagnesaemia and overdose of calcium channel blockers.

Dosage: 0.2 ml kg^{-1} of 10% calcium chloride.

Precautions: Rapid calcium injection may induce bradyarrhythmia and asystole in patients treated with digoxin. The dose should be infused by slow injection via central intravenous access, as calcium may produce chemical burns if it leaks into surrounding tissues.

Magnesium

This is a major intracellular cation and serves as a co-factor in many enzymatic reactions. Magnesium treatment is indicated in children with documented hypomagnesaemia or with polymorphic VT (Torsade de pointes), regardless of cause.

Dosage: 0.5 ml kg^{-1} 10% magnesium sulphate repeated as necessary.

Naloxone

Naloxone is a fast acting (2 minutes after injection) opiate antagonist with duration of action up to 45 minutes. In cases of overdose with drugs such as methadone which has a slow-release form, continuous naloxone infusion may be required to counteract further effects of the opiate.

Indication for use: Symptomatic opiate poisoning. Clinical signs include respiratory depression, coma, miosis, hypotension and decreased perfusion.

Dosage: The recommended initial dose is 100 mcg kg^{-1} in children under 5 years (maximum 2 mg) and 2 mg over 5 years, administered via IV, IO or intramuscular route. If necessary, naloxone can be repeated every 3 minutes.

A continuous naloxone infusion may be used if it is suspected that the patient has received a large amount of opiates. The infusion can range between 10-160 mcg kg^{-1} h^{-1} and is titrated until a satisfactory sustained response is obtained.

Precautions: Serious complications after naloxone treatment are uncommon (< 2%). However, if used for abrupt withdrawal from opiates, severe complications have been described (e.g., seizures, pulmonary oedema, ventricular arrhythmia and hypertension).

Adenosine

Adenosine is an endogenous nucleotide causing atrioventricular block of very short duration. It impairs accessory bundle re-entry at the atrioventricular node (AV). This accessory bundle is responsible for most SVT in children.

Adenosine is rapidly metabolised by red blood cells and its half-life is only 10 seconds. Therefore, it should be injected rapidly and as close to the heart as possible (via a central or upper limb peripheral intravenous route) and immediately followed by a rapid bolus of 0.9% saline.

Side effects (flushing, headache, hypotension, bronchospasm, anxiety and a sense of impending doom) are short-lived, owing to its short half-life.

Indication for use: Adenosine is used in management of SVT as it impairs accessory bundle re-entry at the AV node.

Dosage: 100 mcg kg^{-1} IV or IO bolus (maximum dose 6 mg) is rapidly followed by 3-5 ml of 0.9% saline. The second dose may be doubled (maximum 12 mg). Continuous cardiac monitoring is mandatory.

Precautions: Children treated with theophylline are less sensitive to the effects of adenosine. Adenosine should be used with caution in asthmatics (as it can invoke severe bronchospasm) and children who have undergone a heart transplant.

Key learning points

- Intraosseous access is the circulatory route of choice in cardiorespiratory arrest and decompensated circulatory failure
- Fluid resuscitation starts with 20 ml kg^{-1} boluses
- After each fluid bolus, the child's condition must be reassessed
- The role of medications is secondary to effective ventilation and chest compressions (and, if indicated, defibrillation) in cardiorespiratory arrest
- The main medication used in cardiorespiratory arrest is IV or IO adrenaline, which can be repeated as necessary every 3-5 minutes
- Amiodarone is used in refractory VF or pulseless VT after the 3rd and 5th shock
- Hypoglycaemia and hyperglycaemia should be avoided

Further reading

Sarisoy O, Balaogh K, Tugay S, Barn E, Gokalp AS. Efficacy of magnesium sulphate for treatment of ventricular tachycardia in Amitriptyline overdose Paediatric Emergency care 2007; 23: 9, 646-648.

Dauchot P, Gravenstein JS. Effects of atropine on the electrocardiogram in different age groups. Clin Pharmacol Ther 1971;12:274-80.

Griesdale DE, de Souza RJ, van Dam RM, et al. Intensive insulin therapy and mortality among critically ill patients: a meta-analysis including NICE-SUGAR study data. CMAJ 2009;180:821-7.

Wiener RS, Wiener DC, Larson RJ. Benefits and risks of tight glucose control in critically ill adults: a meta-analysis. JAMA 2008;300:933-44.

Krinsley JS, Grover A. Severe hypoglycemia in critically ill patients: risk factors and outcomes. Crit Care Med 2007;35:2262-7.

Padkin A. Glucose control after cardiac arrest. Resuscitation 2009;80:611-2.

Brenner T, Bernhard M, Helm M et al. Comparison of two Intraosseous systemsfor adult emergency use. Resuscitation 2008; 78: 3, 314-319.

Nadkarni VM, Larkin GL, Peberdy MA, Carey SM, Kaye W, Mancini ME, et al. First documented rhythm and clinical outcome from in-hospital cardiac arrest among children and adults. JAMA. 2006 Jan 4;295(1):50-7.

Finfer S, Bellomo R, Boyce N, French J, Myburgh J, Norton R. A comparison of albumin and saline for fluid resuscitation in the intensive care unit. N Engl J Med. 2004 May 27;350(22):2247-56.

Defibrillation and Cardioversion

CHAPTER 7

Learning outcomes

To understand:

▶ **The indications for defibrillation and cardioversion**

▶ **How to deliver safely an electrical shock using either a manual or automated external defibrillator (AED)**

▶ **The factors influencing the likelihood of successful defibrillation/cardioversion**

Incidence of shockable arrhythmias

Although the initial rhythm in a paediatric cardiorespiratory arrest is far more likely to be asystole or pulseless electrical activity (PEA) than ventricular fibrillation (VF) or pulseless ventricular tachycardia (VT), a shockable rhythm is present in up to 27% of paediatric in-hospital arrests at some point during the resuscitation. When a shockable rhythm is present, the likelihood of a successful outcome is critically dependent on rapid, safe defibrillation.

A defibrillator can be used in the management of a child with circulatory compromise due to VT with a pulse or supraventricular tachycardia (SVT) (Chapter 5). In these situations, the machine is used to perform synchronised DC (direct current) cardioversion which is described in this chapter.

Defibrillation

Defibrillation is the generic term used to describe the procedure of passing an electrical current across the myocardium with the intention of inducing global myocardial depolarisation and restoring organised spontaneous electrical activity. This electrical current may be delivered asynchronously when there is no cardiac output (in VF or pulseless VT), or it may be synchronised with the R wave when there is an output (in SVT or VT with a pulse), the latter being called cardioversion.

The energy dosage should cause minimal myocardial injury. The electrical current delivered to the heart depends on the selected energy (in joules) and the resistance to current flow (thoracic impedance). If the impedance is high, the energy requirement will be increased.

Factors determining thoracic impedance

The factors that potentially affect thoracic impedance and therefore the energy required include:

- defibrillator paddle/pad size
- interface between paddles/pads and the child's skin
- positioning of the paddles/pads on the chest wall
- pressure exerted on the paddles
- chest wall thickness and obesity

Types of defibrillators

Defibrillators are either automatic (i.e. automated external defibrillators) or manually operated. They may be capable of delivering either monophasic or biphasic shocks. Automated external defibrillators (AEDs) are pre-set for all parameters including the energy dose.

Manual defibrillators capable of delivering the full range of energy requirements for newborns through to adults must be available within all healthcare facilities caring for children at risk of cardiorespiratory arrest.

In children requiring cardioversion (e.g. a child with circulatory failure from SVT) a manual defibrillator should be used. An AED cannot be used for cardioversion unless it has a manual mode, but even then the energy level that will be delivered will be greater than that recommended for cardioversion of most children.

Monophasic defibrillators

Monophasic defibrillators are no longer manufactured but may remain in use. They deliver a unipolar (one way) current.

Biphasic defibrillators

There are various types of biphasic waveform but there is no data to support one being superior to another. There is however, good evidence that biphasic defibrillators are more effective than monophasic ones. A biphasic defibrillator delivers a current that flows in a positive direction, and then in reverse for a specified duration. First shock efficacy for long-lasting VF/pulseless VT is better with biphasic than monophasic waveforms. Biphasic waves also appear to cause less post-shock cardiac dysfunction.

Paddles or pads?

Manual defibrillation can be performed using either self-adhesive pads, i.e. 'hands free' defibrillation or the machines paddles.

Rarely manual paddles are used; if they are, separate defibrillation gel pads first need to be applied to the child's chest wall to ensure good contact and reduce transthoracic impedance. These gel pads tend to fall off during chest compressions, often requiring repositioning before each

EUROPEAN PAEDIATRIC LIFE SUPPORT

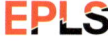

Chapter 7 Defibrillation and Cardioversion

defibrillation attempt. Additionally, they can lead to spurious asystole on ECG analysis as the gel becomes polarised and less effective as a conducting agent on repeated defibrillation attempts. This phenomenon is not encountered with the self-adhesive pads.

Self-adhesive pads are widely used. They are safe, effective and generally preferable to defibrillator paddles. A major advantage of using self-adhesive pads is that they allow the rescuer to defibrillate from a safe distance, rather than having to lean across the patient; this is particularly important when access to the patient is restricted in a confined space. They deliver the shock more rapidly and with less interruption to CPR as the machine can be charged whilst chest compression is in progress.

Position of self-adhesive pads

Self-adhesive pads should be placed on the child's chest in a position that 'brackets' the heart to facilitate the flow of electrical current across it. The standard positioning is to place one pad just below the right clavicle to the right of the sternum and the other in the mid-axillary line on the left of the chest (Figure 7.1).

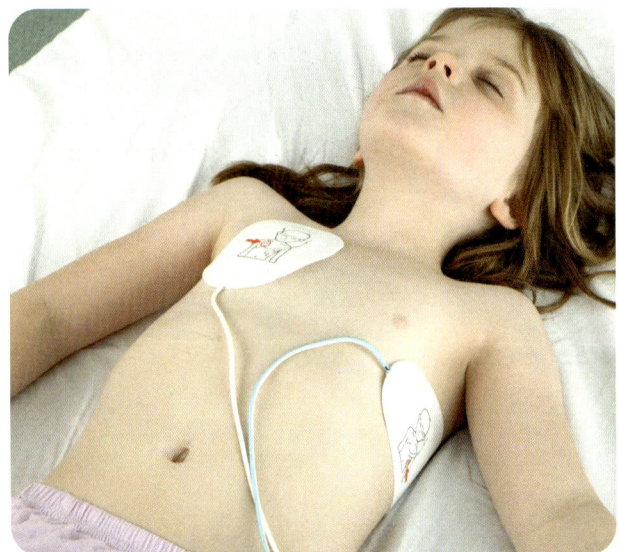

Figure 7.1 Self-adhesive defibrillation pads in position on a child

If using the defibrillator paddles, the aim is to ensure the maximal contact with the chest wall. The largest available paddles should be selected but they must not come in to contact with each other. Generally, the standard (adult) size paddles are appropriate for use in children over 10 kg body weight. If the child is smaller than this, the infant paddles (approximately 4.5 cm diameter) should be used. If infant paddles are unavailable for use on a small child, then the standard paddles can be placed in an anteroposterior (front and back) position instead. When delivering the shock, firm pressure needs to be exerted onto the paddles by the rescuer.

When using self-adhesive pads, it is essential to ensure that they do not touch each other. Selection of appropriate pads relating to the child's size/age may also be necessary, although this varies between manufacturers. The pads should be smoothed onto the child's chest ensuring that no air is trapped underneath as this will increase impedance and reduce the efficiency of the defibrillation shock. Although the pads are generally labelled right and left or have a diagram of their correct positioning on the chest, it does not matter if they have been reversed. Therefore if they have accidentally been placed the wrong way round they should be left in place and not repositioned. Repositioning results in time wasting and the self-adhesive pads may stick less effectively.

Care must be taken when placing defibrillator pads/paddles on children who have an implantable cardioverter-defibrillator (ICD) or cardiac pacemaker, since the current delivered by an external defibrillator may travel along their wire/lead, resulting in burns where they are in contact with the myocardium. Manual defibrillation pads/paddles must be placed at least 12 cm from the pacemaker/ICD site; this may necessitate anteroposterior positioning in some children.

Defibrillation may increase the resistance at the contact point and the 'threshold' for pacing over a period of time. If resuscitation of these children is successful, the pacemaker threshold must be regularly checked for some months after the event.

Energy levels

Manual defibrillators

Manual defibrillators (Figure 7.2) have several advantages over AEDs and therefore must be readily available in all healthcare settings where children at risk of cardiorespiratory arrest may be cared for, even when AEDs are located nearby. The advantages include:

- ability to alter energy levels

- trained operators can diagnose arrhythmias and, when appropriate, deliver shocks more rapidly (with AEDs this diagnosis must await the results of the machine's rhythm analysis)

- additional facilities permit other treatments, e.g. synchronised cardioversion or external pacing

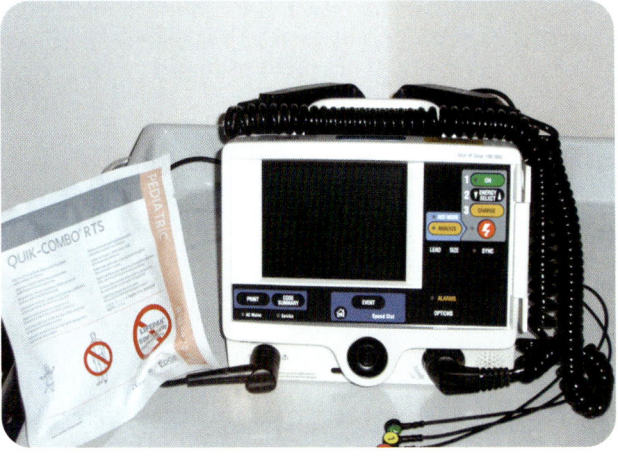

Figure 7.2 Manual defibrillator

When using a manual defibrillator an energy dose of 4 J per kg body weight (4 J kg^{-1}) should be used for all shocks, regardless of whether they are monophasic or biphasic waveforms. In a large child, the adult dosages should not be exceeded, i.e. when using a monophasic machine the maximum dose is 360 J for all shocks, or when using a biphasic machine the maximum for the first shock is 150-200 J. Subsequent energy levels vary depending on the machine used; the manufacturer's guidance should be referred to.

Automated external defibrillators

These machines are now widely available as fully or semi automated devices (Figure 7.3). They are safe, reliable and sophisticated and are increasingly used by health professionals and lay rescuers.

If there is any likelihood of use in infants and small children AED purchasers should check with the manufacturer that the machine is suitable. Machines with paediatric attenuation devices are preferable.

The AED will analyse the patient's ECG rhythm, determine whether a defibrillation shock is indicated and facilitate the delivery of a shock. In the semi-automated models, the shock delivery requires the rescuer to follow the AED prompts and press the relevant button.

Some of the models available to healthcare professionals have the facility for the operator to override the AED and deliver a shock independently of any prompting by the machine.

The main advantages of AEDs are that they recognise specific shockable rhythms and therefore a shock can be delivered by a lay person. They are also relatively cheap and lightweight and have therefore replaced many manual defibrillators. Available AEDs have been tested extensively against libraries of adult ECG rhythms and in trials in adults and children. They are extremely accurate in rhythm recognition in both adults and children.

If a child > 25 kg (approximately 8 years) requires defibrillation, a standard adult AED can be used.

If a child of < 25 kg (or 8 years) requires emergency defibrillation, and there is no manual defibrillator available, an AED can be used. The AED should ideally be equipped with a dose attenuator, which decreases the delivered energy to a lower, more appropriate dosage (generally 50-75 J). If such an AED is unavailable in an emergency situation, then a standard AED with adult energy levels may be used. The upper dose limit for safe defibrillation is unknown but higher doses than the previously recommended 4 J kg^{-1} have defibrillated children effectively and without significant adverse effects. Higher doses are acceptable because defibrillation is the only effective treatment for VF/pulseless VT.

Infants have a much lower incidence of shockable rhythms and good quality CPR is the treatment priority. If an infant is in a shockable rhythm however and a manual machine is not available, use of an AED (preferably with attenuator) may be considered.

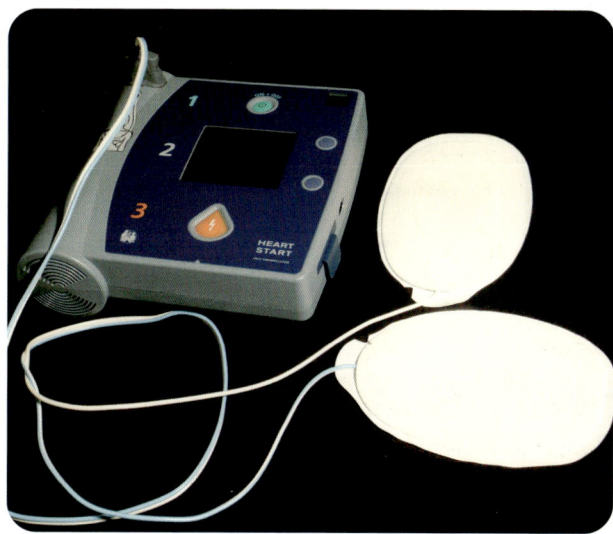

Figure 7.3 An automated external defibrillator

Minimal interruption to chest compression

Every time chest compression is interrupted, even for a brief period, coronary and cerebral perfusion pressure fall and several compressions are needed to return these pressures to their previous levels. Interruptions should therefore be minimised during the defibrillation sequence.

- If a shockable rhythm is still present the defibrillator should be charged whilst chest compressions are continued.

- compressions should be resumed straight after the shock with no check of either the monitor or patient.

Safety issues when undertaking defibrillation

The safety of the rescuers as well as that of the child is paramount. The following factors must be considered:

Oxygen

All free-flowing oxygen delivery devices (O_2 masks or nasal cannulae) must be removed from the immediate area and placed at least one metre from the child. If the child is being ventilated via a tracheal tube, the ventilation bag or ventilator tubing can be left connected if it forms part of a closed circuit. If the circuit is disconnected for whatever reason, the devices must be placed at least one metre away from the child.

Dry surfaces

Any wet clothing should be removed from the immediate area. The surface the child is laid on and the child's chest should be wiped dry if necessary, before shock delivery.

Contact with patient

The person delivering the shock must ensure that neither they nor any other rescuers/relatives are in direct or indirect contact with the child during shock delivery.

There should be no contact between the paddles/ pads and any metal objects (e.g. jewellery) or items such as transdermal medication or diathermy pads.

Operator instructions

Familiarity with the defibrillator being used increases safety and operator efficiency. Operators must also ensure that they issue clear instructions to the rest of the team/bystanders to facilitate safe practice throughout the procedure.

Sequence of actions for manual asynchronous defibrillation

Having confirmed cardiorespiratory arrest, CPR should be commenced (or restarted) while the person delivering the shock prepares as follows:

1. Confirm presence of shockable rhythm (VF/VT) via self-adhesive/monitoring pads or ECG monitor during brief pause in chest compressions

2. Resume chest compressions immediately while designated person applies self-adhesive pads (if not already applied) on the child's chest

3. Plan your actions before pausing CPR for rhythm analysis. Make sure all the team knows the plan before stopping chest compressions

4. The designated person selects the appropriate energy (4 J kg^{-1}) and presses the charge button

5. While the defibrillator is charging warn all rescuers other than the individual performing the chest compressions to "stand clear", and remove any oxygen delivery device as appropriate

6. Once the defibrillator is charged, tell the rescuer doing the chest compressions to "stand clear"; when clear and after confirming continued VF/VT, administer the shock

7. Without reassessing the rhythm or feeling for a pulse, restart CPR starting with chest compressions

8. Continue CPR for 2 minutes; the team leader prepares the team for the next pause in CPR (steps 4 and 5)

9. If VF/VT persists deliver a second shock (as for steps 6 and 7)

Further management of shockable cardiac arrest rhythms is described in Chapter 8.

Considerations when using an AED

The AED pads are placed in the same position as manual defibrillators (Figure 7.1).

Sequence of actions for using an AED

The following guidance should be used with both semi or fully automated AEDs, with or without a paediatric dose attenuating device:

1. Ensure safety of the child and rescuers/bystanders

2. Start BLS. If more than one rescuer is available, one should summon help as appropriate, and then return to assist with BLS and attachment of the AED

   If only one rescuer is available, they should perform one minute of CPR before attaching the AED (unless a cardiac cause is suspected)

3. Switch on the AED and attach self-adhesive pads. If more than one rescuer is present, BLS should be continued whilst the AED is attached

4. Follow the AED prompts

5. Ensure no-one touches the child while the rhythm is being analysed

6. If defibrillation is indicated:
   - Ensure no-one touches the child
   - Press the shock delivery button as directed
   - Continue as directed by the AED prompts

7. If no shock is indicated:
   - Resume BLS immediately
   - Continue as directed by the AED prompts

8. Continue resuscitation until:
   - Help arrives and takes over management
   - The child starts to show 'signs of life'
   - The rescuer becomes too exhausted to continue

NB Do not switch off the AED whilst CPR is continued

Testing the defibrillator

Defibrillators should be regularly tested as per manufacturer and local policies. All potential operators should familiarise themselves with the specific operating procedures of their available machines.

Considerations when undertaking synchronised DC cardioversion

Cardioversion is the timed delivery of an electrical shock from the defibrillator. It is a procedure that can be used in the treatment of symptomatic SVT or VT with a pulse. The delivery of the electric shock is synchronised with the R wave of the ECG to minimise the risk of inducing VF.

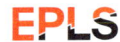

The application of the pads and the safety precautions are the same as for asynchronous defibrillation, but there are some additional considerations. These include:

- **Sedation/anaesthesia** needs to be administered (if the child is conscious) before synchronised cardioversion is performed
- **Synchronisation mode** on the defibrillator must be activated and on some machines it may need to be re-selected if repeat shock(s) are required or if the machine is accidentally turned off between shocks.
- **Increase the ECG gain** to ensure the defibrillator identifies all the R waves on the child's ECG
- **Energy levels** for synchronised cardioversion are lower than for asynchronous defibrillation. The initial dose is 0.5-1 J kg^{-1} although this may be increased to 2 J kg^{-1} if the arrhythmia persists
- **ECG electrodes** are needed for some defibrillators to operate in the synchronised mode
- **Delay in shock delivery** can occur between the operator depressing the delivery button(s) and the actual shock being delivered. This is because the machine will only deliver the shock when it identifies an R wave. In practice it means that the operator must keep the shock delivery button(s) depressed until this occurs

Following cardioversion, some defibrillators may remain in the synchronised mode which is a potential risk; a defibrillator left in the synchronised mode will not be immediately ready to deliver a shock to treat a VF/pulseless VT cardiorespiratory arrest victim, therefore always leave the defibrillator in the non-synchronised mode.

Key learning points

- Shockable rhythms may occur in up to 27% of in-hospital resuscitation attempts in children
- For the child in VF/pulseless VT, defibrillation (as early as possible) is the only effective means of restoring a spontaneous circulation
- Modern biphasic defibrillators have a high first shock efficacy; use single shocks at 4 J kg^{-1} interspersed with 2 minutes CPR
- Chest compressions should be interrupted as little as possible
- A standard adult AED can be used for children > 25 kg
- An AED that can specifically recognise paediatric shockable arrhythmias and that is equipped with a dose attenuator is preferred for children < 25 kg

Further reading

Atkinson E, Mikysa B et al. Specificity and sensitivity of automated external defibrillator rhythm analysis in infants and children. Ann Emerg Med 2003;42: 185-96.

Benson D, Jr., Smith W, Dunnigan A, Sterba R, Gallagher J. Mechanisms of regular wide QRS tachycardia in infants and children. Am J Cardiol 1982;49:1778-88.

Berg RA, Chapman FW et al. Attenuated adult biphasic shocks compared with weight-based monophasic shocks in a swine model of prolonged pediatric ventricular fibrillation. Resuscitation 2004; 61: 189-197.

Berg RA, Samson RA et al. Better outcome after pediatric defibrillation dosage than adult dosage in a swine model of pediatric ventricular fibrillation. J Am Coll Cardiol 2005;45: 786-9.

Clark CB, Zhang Y et al. Pediatric transthoracic defibrillation: biphasic versus monophasic waveforms in an experimental model. Resuscitation 2001;51: 159-63.

Edelson DP, Abella BS, Kramer-Johansen J, et al. Effects of compression depth and pre-shock pauses predict defibrillation failure during cardiac arrest. Resuscitation 2006;71:137-45.

Eftestol T, Sunde K, Steen PA. Effects of interrupting precordial compressions on the calculated probability of defibrillation success during out-of-hospital cardiac arrest. Circulation 2002;105:2270-3.

Faddy SC, Powell J et al. Biphasic and monophasic shocks for transthoracic defibrillation: A meta analysis of randomised controlled trials. Resuscitation 2003;8: 9-16.

Jorgenson D, Morgan C, Snyder D et al. Energy attenuator for pediatric application of an automated external defibrillator. Crit Care Med 2002;30:S145-7.

Rossano JQ, Schiff L, Kenney MA, Atkins DL. Survival is not correlated with defibrillation dosing in pediatric out-of-hospital ventricular fibrillation. Circulation 2003;108: IV-320-321.

Seeram N, Wren C. Supraventricular tachycardia in infants: response to initial treatment. Arch Dis Child 1990;65:127-9.

Samson R, Berg R et al. Use of automated external defibrillators for children: an update. An advisory statement from the Pediatric Advanced Life Support Task Force, International Liaison Committee on Resuscitation. Resuscitation 2003;57: 237-43.

Schneider T, Martens PR et al. Multicenter, randomized, controlled trial of 150-J biphasic shocks compared with 200- to 360-J monophasic shocks in the resuscitation of out-of-hospital cardiac arrest victims. Circulation 2000;102: 1780-1787.

Chapter 7 Defibrillation and Cardioversion

Management of Cardiorespiratory Arrest

CHAPTER 8

Learning outcomes

To understand:

- How to continue resuscitation until experienced help arrives
- The management of non-shockable cardiac arrest rhythms
- The management of shockable cardiac arrest rhythms
- The potentially reversible causes of cardiorespiratory arrest
- Considerations of when to stop resuscitation attempts

Resuscitation process

The division between basic life support (BLS) and advanced life support (ALS) is somewhat artificial. Resuscitation is a continuous process, and the elements of effective BLS must be continued until return of a spontaneous circulation (ROSC), even when experienced help arrives (i.e. the EMS or clinical emergency team) and appropriate equipment can be used to facilitate delivery of advanced techniques.

All clinical staff within a healthcare facility should be able to:

- immediately recognise cardiorespiratory arrest
- start appropriate resuscitation (BLS with available adjuncts as per local policy)
- summon the clinical emergency team using the standard telephone number (2222 in-hospital) and/or EMS (via national 999 or 112 system)

The exact sequence of actions will be dependent on several factors including:

- Location of event (clinical or non-clinical area)
- Number of first responders
- Skills of first responders
- Availability of resuscitation equipment
- Local policies

Location of event

Clinical area

If the child is seriously ill on a ward, it is likely that they will have been deteriorating over a period of time. Many wards now employ an 'early warning scoring system' based on physiological parameters, which is designed to identify seriously ill children before they become decompensated; experienced staff are alerted and can initiate appropriate management strategies to prevent cardiorespiratory arrest occurring.

When a child does suffer a cardiorespiratory arrest in a clinical area, appropriate resuscitation equipment and trained staff should be readily available.

Non-clinical area

There may be occasions when a child suffers a cardiorespiratory arrest in a non-clinical area (e.g. corridors, car park, play area). In these areas, there may not be readily available equipment or trained staff, and these children may have a more prolonged period of BLS before help arrives.

The guidance in the first section of this chapter is primarily aimed at healthcare professionals who may be an initial responder in a clinical emergency situation and have rapid access to resuscitation equipment. The guidance in the second section of this chapter is primarily aimed at the team providing experienced help including guidance for the team leader.

Number of first responders

A single rescuer must not leave the collapsed child, but should start appropriate resuscitation (e.g. BLS or BLS with BMV) and ensure that further help is summoned. If the condition is thought to be due to a primary cardiac cause EMS help is activated before BLS has started. Within a clinical area, there are usually more staff nearby who can be alerted, either by the first responder shouting for help and/or using an emergency call button system. As soon as a second rescuer arrives, they should be sent to summon further assistance in line with local policy (i.e. activate the clinical emergency team). On their return (or the arrival of other staff) simultaneous interventions can be undertaken, according to the skills of the available staff.

Skills of first responders

All healthcare providers should be able to recognise cardiorespiratory arrest, shout for help and start resuscitation to the level to which they have been trained.

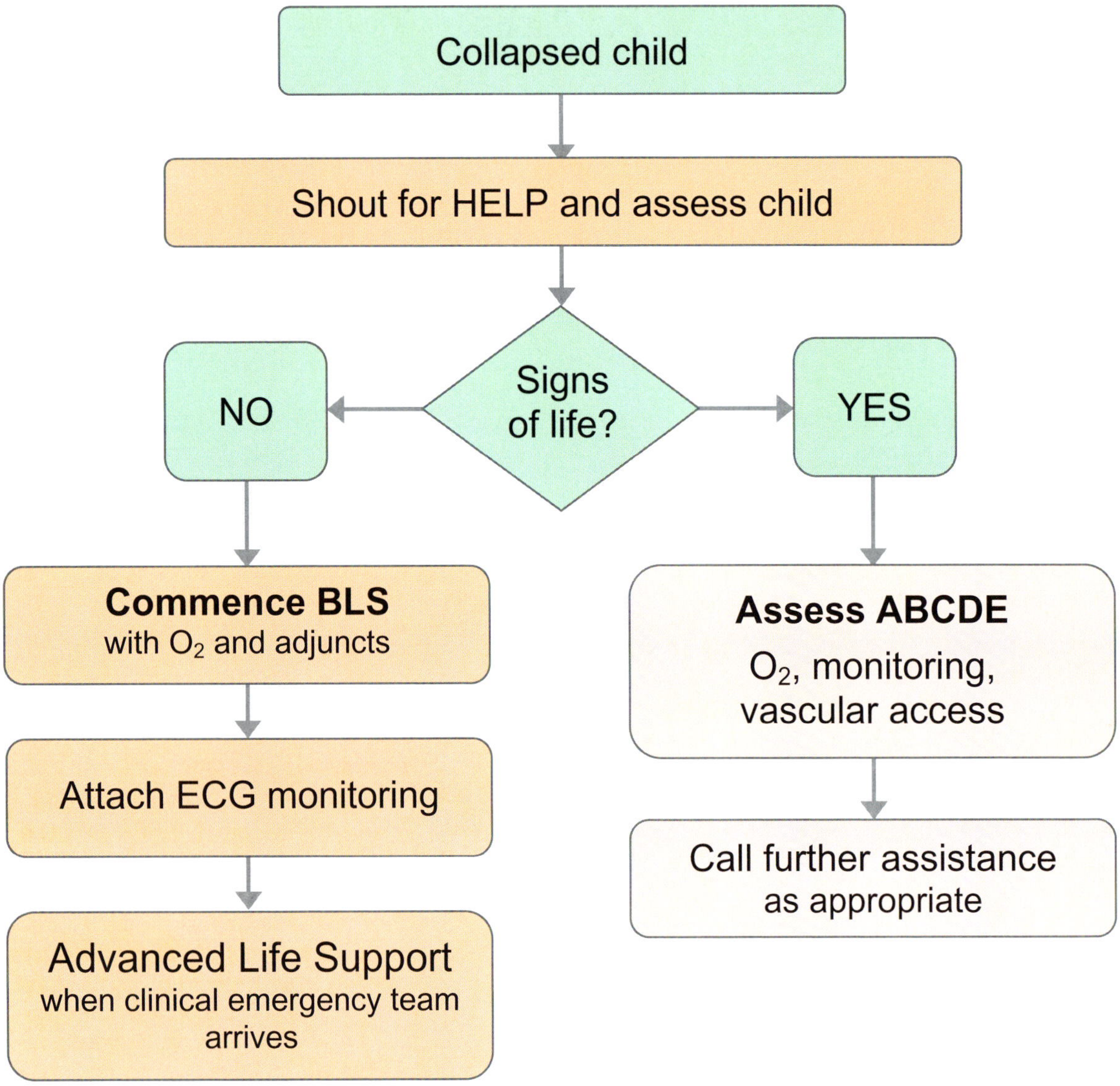

Chapter 8 Management of Cardiorespiratory Arrest

```
                    Collapsed child
                           │
                           ▼
              Shout for HELP and assess child
                           │
                           ▼
                     Signs of life?
                    ╱             ╲
                  NO               YES
                  │                 │
                  ▼                 ▼
           Commence BLS        Assess ABCDE
         with O₂ and adjuncts  O₂, monitoring,
                  │            vascular access
                  ▼                 │
         Attach ECG monitoring      ▼
                  │           Call further assistance
                  ▼              as appropriate
        Advanced Life Support
        when clinical emergency
              team arrives
```

Figure 8.1 Initial resuscitation management

Staff will have been trained to different levels according to local policies; some may only undertake BLS, whilst others would be expected to undertake additional techniques to manage airway, breathing and circulation. First responders should only undertake the skills they have been trained to perform; their initial priority in paediatric cardiorespiratory arrest should be to ensure effective ventilation and oxygenation with good quality BLS. As more experienced help arrives, other interventions can be undertaken.

Availability of resuscitation equipment

All clinical areas where children are likely to be cared for should be equipped with resuscitation equipment to help with the management of a clinical emergency. The staff in each area should have responsibility for maintenance and regular checking of this clinical emergency equipment, as this will facilitate their familiarity with it. By employing standardised resuscitation equipment hospital-wide, the clinical emergency team should also know exactly what equipment is readily available to them when called to deal with a child in any area.

Local policies

As well as specifying the levels of resuscitation skills for different staff groups, hospitals should also have policies regarding the composition of, and calling criteria for, their clinical emergency teams. In some centres, there might be more than one emergency team (dictated by the geographical layout or the clinical specialties of the hospital) or there may be different types of team (e.g. a cardiac arrest team and a medical emergency team). Staff must be aware of their local systems and trained to act accordingly.

These operational issues should be audited. They can be practised (and their effectiveness measured) by undertaking 'mock' emergency calls.

In-hospital cardiorespiratory arrest sequence

The initial management of an apparently collapsed child is summarised in Figure 8.1.

Safety

The approach described in Chapter 3 should be followed to ensure firstly the safety of the rescuers and then that of the child. Whilst the risk of contracting infection is low, personal protective measures should be employed as soon as practicable (e.g. gloves, aprons, eye protection, face masks). In situations where the child may have a severe infection (e.g. open TB, Swine flu or SARS) rescuers must be equipped with full protective measures. In areas where such children may be treated, this equipment should be immediately available.

Stimulate

The approach described in Chapter 3 should be followed to establish the responsiveness of an apparently unconscious child.

Responsive child

If the child responds (i.e. they demonstrate 'signs of life'), their ABCDE should be assessed. Appropriate interventions should be initiated and further relevant assistance summoned.

Unresponsive child

If the child is unresponsive (i.e. they do not demonstrate 'signs of life'), BLS must be started immediately whilst simultaneously shouting for more assistance.

Shout

The single rescuer must not leave the child but shout loudly for help and start BLS, using basic airway adjuncts and BMV if they are immediately available. It would also be appropriate for them to activate a bedside emergency call button system if this is available.

If there is a second rescuer available they should be sent to summon more assistance, and return to help with the resuscitation attempt. If there is resuscitation equipment nearby, they should bring this to the bedside, but this must not delay calling the clinical emergency team.

Airway

The airway should be opened as described in Chapter 3. If there is suction available, it may be necessary to use this to clear any secretions in the upper airway before proceeding to ventilation.

Breathing

If the child is not breathing, or only gasping ineffectively, initial rescue breaths should be delivered by the most appropriate method available (e.g. expired air rescue breaths with a barrier device or self-inflating bag-mask device with supplemental oxygen).

If there are two rescuers available and at least one is trained in the use of BMV, the rescuer managing the airway and delivering the rescue breaths should be positioned behind the child's head. A second rescuer should be positioned at the side of the child to perform chest compressions if indicated.

Circulation

Assessment

If a child, who is not breathing adequately, does not respond quickly to rescue breaths, they are unlikely to have an adequate spontaneous circulation. However, in the hospital setting, it is appropriate for a rescuer to briefly try and determine the presence of a central pulse whilst simultaneously observing for 'signs of life'.

If an adequate pulse (i.e. > 60 min^{-1}) is DEFINITELY felt, but breathing is absent or inadequate, the child's airway must be maintained and rescue breathing continued at a rate of 12-20 min^{-1}.

If the child's pulse is absent or inadequate (i.e. < 60 min^{-1}), or there is any doubt and there are no other 'signs of life', chest compressions must be started.

Rhythm recognition

As soon as resuscitation equipment is available, the emphasis is on ensuring that effective CPR is enhanced by BMV with supplemental oxygen. The next step is to establish the child's cardiac rhythm, and therefore an ECG monitor or defibrillator must be attached. The priority is deciding whether the cardiac rhythm is shockable or not, in order to determine the ongoing management of the cardiorespiratory arrest. If an AED is used, the machine will guide the rescuers through the appropriate sequence of actions. However, in paediatric areas of a hospital, it is often an ECG monitor that is most readily available and therefore the clinical emergency team members must be able to rapidly identify whether they are dealing with a child in a shockable or non-shockable rhythm.

Shockable or non-shockable cardiac rhythms

In children, the most common initial cardiorespiratory arrest rhythms are non-shockable, i.e. profound bradycardia, asystole or pulseless electrical activity (PEA).

The shockable cardiorespiratory arrest rhythms, i.e. ventricular fibrillation (VF) and pulseless ventricular tachycardia (VT) are less common. When these occur, it is often in a child with underlying cardiac disease.

The management of shockable and non-shockable cardiorespiratory arrest is outlined in the paediatric advanced life support algorithm (Figure 8.2).

Non-shockable rhythms (asystole and PEA)

Asystole

This rhythm is characterised by the total absence of effective electrical and mechanical activity in the heart (Figure 8.3).

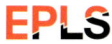

Chapter 8 Management of Cardiorespiratory Arrest

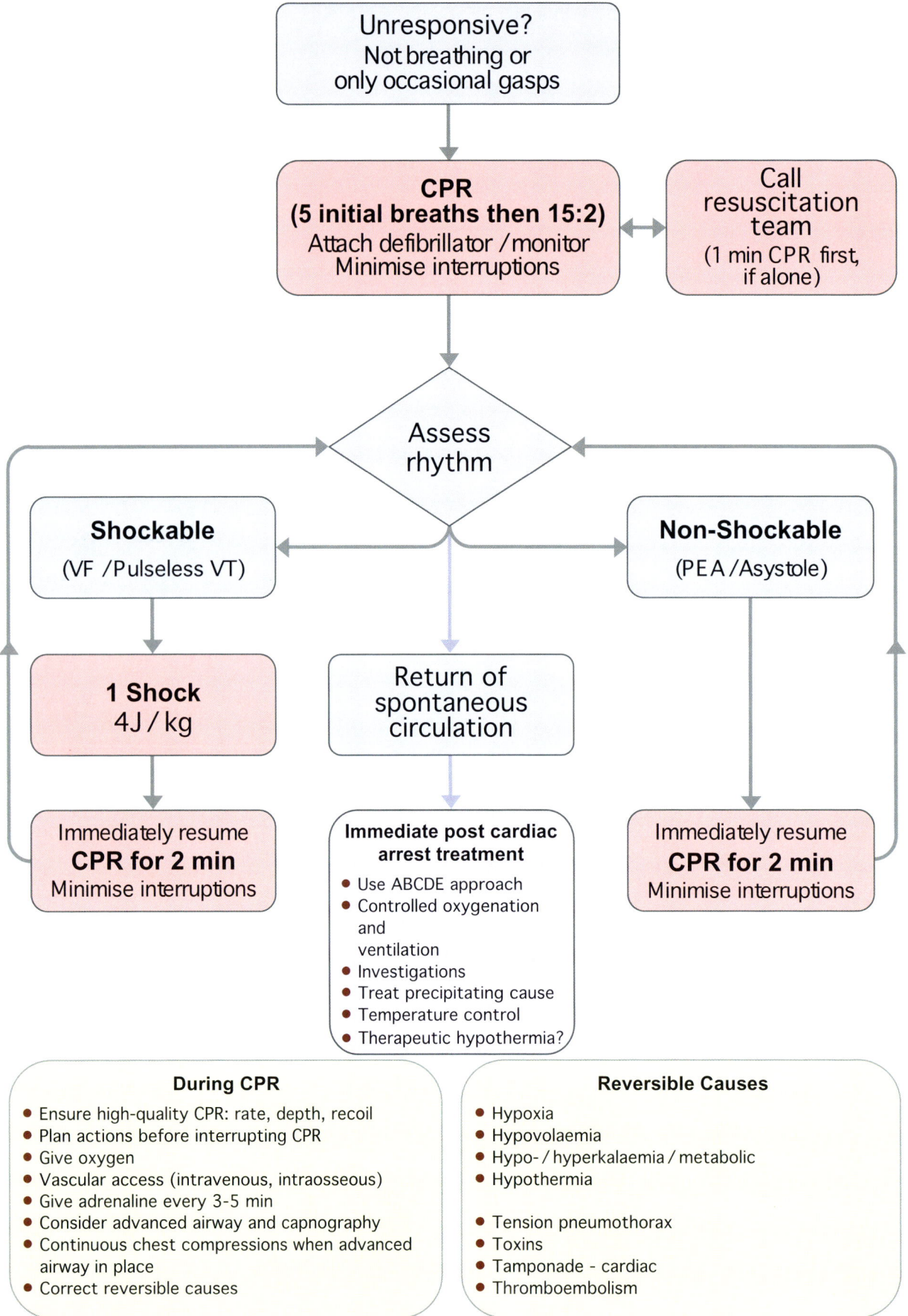

Figure 8.2 Paediatric advanced life support algorithm

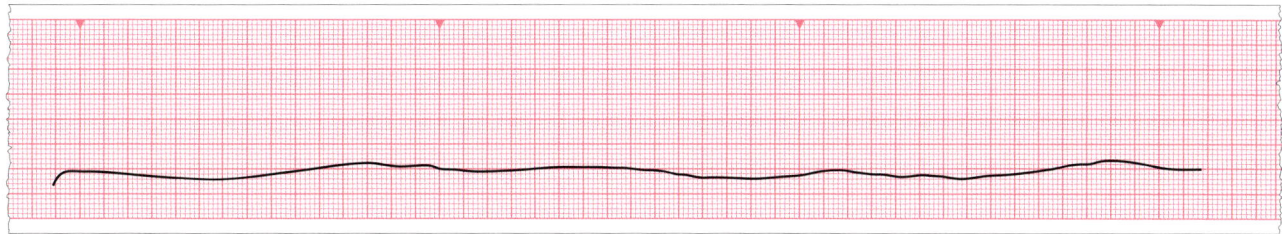

Figure 8.3 Asystole

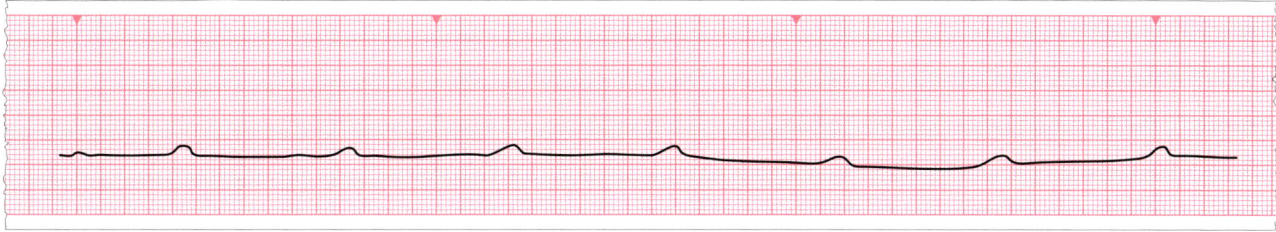

Figure 8.4 P-wave asystole

It can be simulated by artefact (e.g. detached ECG leads/electrodes) so it is important to quickly check the equipment. In asystole, there is no ventricular function, but occasionally there is some residual atrial activity, which may be seen on the ECG as P waves (Figure 8.4). It is often preceded by severe bradycardia. The most common cause of bradycardia in a child is hypoxia but hypotension, hypothermia or hypoglycaemia can depress normal cardiac activity and slow conduction through cardiac tissues.

Pulseless Electrical Activity (PEA)

This rhythm is defined as organised cardiac electrical activity in the absence of a palpable central pulse. It is thought that some of these children may have some myocardial contraction, but it is too weak and ineffective to produce a detectable pulse or blood pressure. The ECG rhythm displayed is often a slow, broad complex one, although any variation of regular QRS complexes may be seen.

All the cardiac arrest rhythms, but particularly PEA, may be due to an underlying reversible condition (see below); it is essential that any treatable causes are identified and managed.

Management of asystole and PEA

- **Perform continuous CPR:**
    - Continue to ventilate with high-concentration oxygen.
    - If ventilating with bag-mask give 15 chest compressions to 2 ventilations.
    - Use a compression rate of 100-120 min^{-1}.
    - If the patient is intubated, chest compressions can be continuous as long as this does not interfere with satisfactory ventilation.
    - Once the child has been intubated and compressions are uninterrupted use a ventilation rate of approximately 10-12 min^{-1}.

- **Give adrenaline:**
    - If IV or IO access has been established, give adrenaline 10 mcg kg^{-1} (0.1 ml kg^{-1} of 1 in 10,000 solution).
    - If there is no circulatory access, obtain IO access.
    - If circulatory access is not present, and cannot be quickly obtained, but the patient has a tracheal tube in place, consider giving adrenaline 100 mcg kg^{-1} via the tracheal tube. This is the least satisfactory route.

- **Continue CPR, only pausing briefly every 2 minutes to check for rhythm change.**

- Give adrenaline 10 mcg kg^{-1} every 3 to 5 minutes, (i.e. every other loop), while continuing to maintain effective chest compression and ventilation without interruption.
    - **Consider and correct reversible causes:** (4Hs & 4Ts) page 72.

If, during the rhythm check, organised electrical activity is seen on the monitor, check for 'signs of life' and a central pulse:

- If a pulse > 60 min^{-1} and/or 'signs of life' are present, start post-resuscitation care
- If there is no pulse, or you are unsure, and there are no 'signs of life' (i.e. PEA) continue with 'non-shockable' algorithm

If the cardiac rhythm changes to VF or pulseless VT, the rescuers must change their management to follow the shockable side of the paediatric advanced life support algorithm (Figure 8.2).

Chapter 8 Management of Cardiorespiratory Arrest

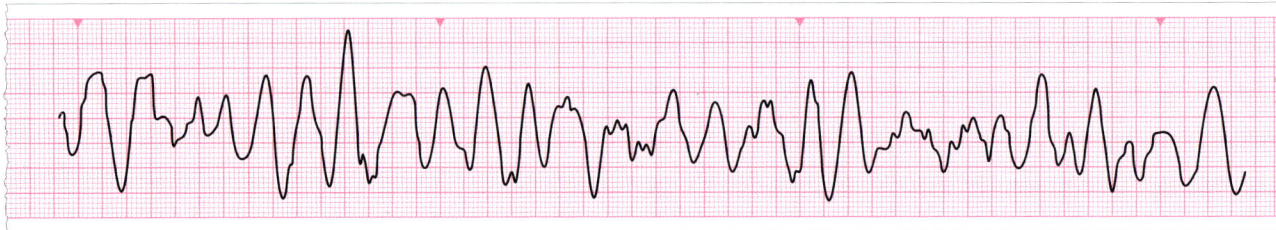

Figure 8.5 Coarse ventricular fibrillation

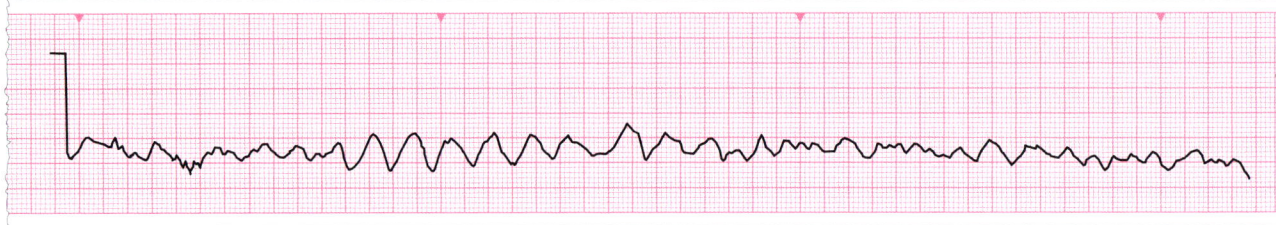

Figure 8.6 Fine ventricular fibrillation

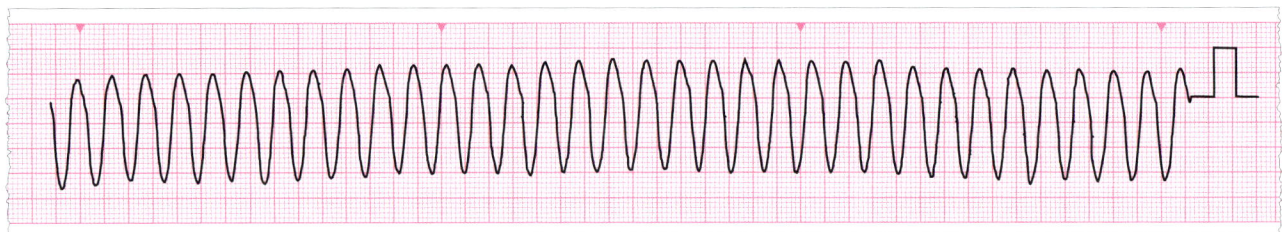

Figure 8.7 Ventricular tachycardia

Shockable rhythms (VF and pulseless VT)

Ventricular fibrillation

This rhythm shows rapid, chaotic, irregular waves of varying frequency and amplitude. VF is sometimes classified as 'coarse or fine' depending on the amplitude (height) of the complexes (Figures 8.5 and 8.6). When there is doubt as to whether a rhythm is fine VF or asystole, rescuers should not deliver a defibrillation shock but should continue with CPR. It is unlikely that fine VF will be successfully shocked into a perfusing rhythm, but continuing good quality CPR may increase the frequency and amplitude of the VF and improve the chances of successful defibrillation, i.e to produce a perfusing rhythm. If the cardiac rhythm is clearly VF, defibrillation should be performed without delay.

Pulseless VT

This rhythm is a broad complex tachycardia (Figure 8.7). It is rare in children and is managed in the same way as VF, i.e. defibrillation.

Management of VF and pulseless VT

- Continue CPR with BMV and supplemental O_2 until a defibrillator is available
  - **Defibrillate the heart:**
  - Charge the defibrillator while another rescuer continues chest compressions.

- Once the defibrillator is charged, pause the chest compressions, quickly ensure that all rescuers are clear of the patient and then deliver the shock. The shock may be delivered by the person doing compressions or another rescuer. This should be planned before stopping compressions.

  - Give 1 shock of 4 J kg^{-1} if using a manual defibrillator.
  - If using an AED for a child > 8 years, use the adult shock energy.
  - If using an AED for a child < 8 years, deliver a paediatric-attenuated adult shock energy.
  (*If neither an attenuated AED or a manual defibrillator are available, use an adult AED*).

- **Resume CPR:**
  - Without reassessing the rhythm or feeling for a pulse, resume CPR **immediately**, starting with chest compression.
  - Consider and correct reversible causes (4Hs and 4Ts)

- **Continue CPR for 2 minutes, then pause briefly to check the monitor:**

- **If still VF/VT, give a second shock** (with same energy level and strategy for delivery as the first shock).

- **Resume CPR**
    - Without reassessing the rhythm or feeling for a pulse, resume CPR **immediately**, starting with chest compression

- **Continue CPR for 2 minutes, then pause briefly to check the monitor**

- **If still VF/VT, give a third shock** (with same energy level and strategy for delivery as the previous shock)

- **Resume CPR**
    - Without reassessing the rhythm or feeling for a pulse, resume CPR **immediately**, starting with chest compression.
    - Give adrenaline 10 mcg kg^{-1} and amiodarone 5 mg kg^{-1} after the 3rd shock, once chest compressions have resumed.
    - Repeat adrenaline every alternate cycle (i.e. every 3-5 minutes) until return of spontaneous circulation (ROSC)
    - Repeat amiodarone 5 mg kg^{-1} one further time, after the 5th shock if still in a shockable rhythm.
    - Continue giving shocks every 2 minutes, continuing compressions during charging of the defibrillator and minimising the breaks in chest compression as much as possible.
    - **Consider and correct reversible causes** (4Hs and 4Ts)

Note: **After each 2 minutes of uninterrupted CPR, pause briefly to assess the rhythm.**

- **If still VF/VT:**
    - Continue CPR with the shockable (VF/VT) sequence.
- **If asystole:**
    - Continue CPR and switch to the non-shockable (asystole or pulseless electrical activity) sequence as above.
- **If organised electrical activity is seen**, check for signs of life and a pulse:
    - If a pulse of > 60 min^{-1} and/or 'signs of life' are present, start post-resuscitation care
    - If there is **no** pulse (or a pulse of < 60 min^{-1}), and there are no other signs of life, continue CPR and continue as for the non-shockable sequence above.

If defibrillation was successful but VF/VT recurs, resume the CPR sequence and defibrillate. Give an amiodarone bolus (unless 2 doses have already been given) and start a continuous infusion.

Rationale for sequence of actions on shockable side of algorithm

- The interval between stopping chest compressions and delivering a shock must be minimal (< 10 seconds); longer interruptions to chest compressions reduce the likelihood of a shock restoring a perfusing rhythm

- Chest compressions are resumed immediately after a shock without reassessing the rhythm or feeling for a pulse because, even if the defibrillation attempt is successful in restoring a rhythm, it is unlikely that the heart will immediately pump effectively. Even if a perfusing rhythm has been restored, giving chest compressions does not increase the chance of VF recurring

If an organised rhythm is observed during a 2 minute cycle of CPR, do not interrupt chest compressions to palpate a pulse, unless the patient shows signs of life demonstrating return of spontaneous circulation (ROSC).

If there is any doubt about the presence of a pulse in a patient who has an organised cardiac rhythm compatible with cardiac output, but no other signs of life, resume CPR for a further 2 minutes.

Ongoing resuscitation

Outcome in all resuscitation attempts is dependent on good quality chest compressions and ventilation (plus defibrillation when indicated for shockable arrhythmias). Performing chest compression is tiring, and to reduce fatigue and maximise efficiency, the rescuer delivering chest compressions should share the work with another by alternating every 2 minutes. As soon as the airway is secured with a tracheal tube, chest compressions should be performed continuously unless this compromises delivery of adequate tidal volumes.

Airway and ventilation

The vast majority of children can be adequately ventilated with BMV in the initial stages of resuscitation; it is often better to continue with this until ROSC rather than attempt tracheal intubation and temporarily interrupt oxygenation during laryngoscopy. However, once the expertise is available, tracheal intubation provides the most reliable airway and will be essential in the post-resuscitation management of a child who has suffered cardiorespiratory arrest.

If laryngoscopy is to be performed during CPR, it should be attempted without interruption of chest compressions, although there may need to be a brief pause as the tracheal tube is passed through the vocal cords.

Following tracheal intubation and confirmation of the correct tube position, it should be secured and then chest compressions can be delivered continuously without a pause for ventilation. Breaths should be delivered at a rate of approximately 10-12 min^{-1}.

Circulatory access

If the child does not already have secure circulatory access, this should be achieved as soon as possible after establishing effective CPR during a cardiorespiratory arrest. The emergency route of choice is intraosseous (Chapter 6).

History and reversible causes

Obtaining relevant information about the child's underlying medical condition and any pre-disposing events can be useful in determining likely causes of, and potential outcome from, the cardiorespiratory arrest.

Any possible causes (or aggravating factors) that have specific treatment must be considered during all cardiorespiratory arrests. The most likely of these can be recalled by the mnemonic '4 Hs and 4 Ts':

> ### The 4 Hs
> 1. **Hypoxia**
> 2. **Hypovolaemia**
> 3. **Hypo/hyperkalaemia/metabolic**
> 4. **Hypothermia**
>
> ### The 4 Ts
> 1. **Tension pneumothorax**
> 2. **Tamponade (cardiac)**
> 3. **Toxins**
> 4. **Thromboembolism**

Hypoxia

This is a frequent cause of paediatric cardiorespiratory arrest. The risks of it occurring, or persisting, during resuscitation should be minimised by ensuring effective ventilation with 100% oxygen. It is essential to ensure that there is adequate, bilateral chest movement. The mnemonic DOPES described in Chapter 4 should be considered in intubated children.

Hypovolaemia

Loss of circulating volume can often result in cardiorespiratory arrest. Hypovolaemia may be due to many different causes (e.g. haemorrhage from trauma, diarrhoea and vomiting, anaphylaxis, severe sepsis) and these need to be identified and treated appropriately. Start rapid circulatory volume replacement with an initial 20 ml kg^{-1} bolus of 0.9% saline solution. Further fluid boluses should be given as described in Chapter 6.

Hypo/hyperkalaemia/metabolic

Electrolyte and metabolic disorders may be suggested by the child's medical history and/or biochemical tests. Specific treatment should be given to correct these problems. An estimation of blood glucose level should be obtained early; both hypo and hyperglycaemia are common and associated with increased morbidity and mortality.

Hypothermia

Low body temperature may be an unlikely problem in hospitalised children, but it should always be considered, particularly in small or premature infants, or in children being managed in the Emergency department. A low-reading thermometer should be used to record a core temperature when hypothermia is considered a possibility.

Tension pneumothorax

Signs of tension pneumothorax (e.g. decreased chest movement and air entry, hyper-resonance on the affected side, tracheal deviation away from the affected side) should be sought, particularly in children who have suffered trauma or following thoracic surgery. If a tension pneumothorax is thought to be present, rapid needle decompression is required, followed by chest drain insertion (page 94).

Tamponade (cardiac)

This is not a common cause of cardiorespiratory arrest in children, but may occur following cardiothoracic surgery, penetrating chest trauma or some viral illnesses. It can be difficult to diagnose as typical signs (e.g. distended neck veins and hypovolaemia) are often masked by the cardiorespiratory arrest. If there is a strong history, needle pericardiocentesis is indicated.

Toxins

In the absence of a confirmed history, accidental or deliberate poisoning with toxins (therapeutic or toxic substances) may only be discovered after laboratory analysis. Appropriate antidotes should be administered as soon as possible when indicated and available, but frequently management of these children is based on measures to support their vital organs. Check the patient's drug chart.

Thromboembolism

It is unusual for children to suffer from thromboembolic complications, but they can occur. If it is considered that this is a cause, appropriate thrombolysis would be needed.

Stopping resuscitation

Resuscitation efforts are unlikely to be successful in achieving ROSC if there have been no signs of cardiac output, despite at least 20 minutes of continuous, good quality CPR in children. In the newborn, withdrawal may be considered after 10 minutes (Chapter 13).

However, it would be appropriate to prolong resuscitation attempts in children with the following conditions:

- hypothermia
- poisoning
- persistent VF/pulseless VT

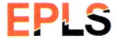

The resuscitation team may also consider that specific circumstances (e.g. awaiting arrival of family members) make it appropriate to maintain resuscitation efforts.

Presence of parents during resuscitation

The opportunity to be present during at least part of the resuscitation of their child should be offered to parents/carers. Evidence suggests that this aids with their grieving process (less anxiety and depression when assessed several months later).

The following points (which apply whether the parent is actually in the room beside their child, or elsewhere in the ward/department) should be considered:

- a specific member of staff should be delegated to remain with the parents throughout to offer empathetic, but realistic, support

- if necessary, an appropriate interpreter must be present to facilitate accuracy of communication between parents and the resuscitation team leader

- physical contact with their child and the opportunity to say 'goodbye' (in unsuccessful resuscitation attempts) should be encouraged

- the resuscitation team leader decides when to stop resuscitation efforts, and not the parents

- a debriefing session for all staff involved should be arranged to offer support and reflect on practice

- appropriate referrals and counselling should be organised for the parents to ensure they receive adequate support

Key learning points

▸ The optimal management of in-hospital cardiorespiratory arrest is always based on the rapid initiation of effective ventilation, oxygenation and chest compression, i.e. ABCDE principles

▸ The paediatric advanced life support algorithm provides a framework for cardiorespiratory arrest management of all children

▸ Asystole and PEA are non-shockable arrhythmias and their management is based on effective CPR, adrenaline administration and treatment of reversible causes

▸ VF and pulseless VT are shockable arrhythmias and their management is based on effective CPR, early defibrillation and treatment of reversible causes

▸ The parents/carers should be supported and, ideally, be present during the resuscitation of their child

Further reading

ILCOR 2010 worksheets on resuscitation
www.americanheart.org/presenter.jhtml?identifier=3060115
References to the basis for resuscitation including the presence of relatives in the resuscitation room are available from this website.

Duncan HP, Frew E: Short-term health system costs of paediatric in-hospital acute life-threatening events including cardiac arrest. Resuscitation 2009;80:529-534.

Edwards ED, Mason BW, Oliver A, Powell CV: Cohort study to test the predictability of the melbourne criteria for activation of the medical emergency team. Arch Dis Child 2010.

Eppich WJ, Brannen M, Hunt EA: Team training: Implications for emergency and critical care pediatrics. Curr Opin Pediatr 2008;20:255-260.

Hanson CC, Randolph GD, Erickson JA, Mayer CM, et al. A reduction in cardiac arrests and duration of clinical instability after implementation of a paediatric rapid response system. Postgrad Med J 2010;86:314-318.

Nolan JP, Soar J, Zideman DA, Biarent D et al. European Resuscitation Council Guidelines for Resuscitation 2010 Section 1. Executive summary. Resuscitation. 2010;81:1219-76.

Thomas EJ, Williams AL, Reichman EF, Lasky RE, et al. Team training in the neonatal resuscitation program for interns: Teamwork and quality of resuscitations. Pediatrics 2010;125:539-546.

Tibballs J, Kinney S: Reduction of hospital mortality and of preventable cardiac arrest and death on introduction of a pediatric medical emergency team. Pediatr Crit Care Med 2009;10:306-312.

Topjian AA, Nadkarni VM, Berg RA: Cardiopulmonary resuscitation in children. Curr Opin Crit Care 2009;15:203-208.

Van Voorhis KT, Willis TS: Implementing a pediatric rapid response system to improve quality and patient safety. Pediatr Clin North Am 2009;56:919-933.

Weinstock P, Halamek LP: Teamwork during resuscitation. Pediatr Clin North Am 2008;55:1011-1024, xi-xii.

Winberg H, Nilsson K, Aneman A: Paediatric rapid response systems: A literature review. Acta Anaesthesiol Scand 2008;52:890-896.

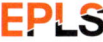

Principles of Post-resuscitation Care

CHAPTER 9

Learning outcomes

To understand:

▸ **The importance of post-resuscitation stabilisation and optimisation of organ function following cardiorespiratory arrest**

▸ **The specific investigations and monitoring indicated**

▸ **How to facilitate the safe transfer of the seriously ill child**

Continued resuscitation

Post-resuscitation care begins when the child has a return of spontaneous circulation (ROSC); however this is merely the first step in the continuous process of resuscitation management. The ultimate goal is to achieve a state of stable haemodynamic and cerebral function, and prevent secondary organ damage.

Secondary organ damage includes:

- Hypoxic-ischaemic brain injury
- Ischaemic myocardial damage
- Hypoxic pulmonary damage
- Acute renal failure
- Coagulopathy
- Ischaemic hepatitis
- Acute gastro-intestinal lesions

The ABCDE approach must also be followed in the immediate post-resuscitation phase as it focuses management priorities. However, the ongoing care of the child requires the expertise of many healthcare professionals and is best delivered in a PICU facility. This may require a specialist team to facilitate an optimal safe transfer.

Stabilisation of airway and breathing

The aim of respiratory management is to maintain adequate oxygenation and ventilation, avoiding hypoxia and hypo/hypercapnia, which may worsen the child's prognosis.

If the child has been resuscitated using BMV a decision needs to be made whether the child or infant will need ongoing ventilation and placement of a tracheal tube. Factors that may affect this decision include:

- unsecured airway
- requirement for the safe transfer to a PICU
- conscious level (AVPU) at level P or less means that there will be no protective airway reflexes
- lung pathology resulting in a need for positive pressure ventilation

BMV causes gastric distention which will impede ventilation and may cause vomiting. A gastric tube is usually required to deflate the stomach if it has become distended following BMV.

Children and infants who remain intubated and ventilated will need sedation and analgesia in most cases.

Following intubation, the most common post-resuscitation airway/breathing complications can be identified by considering the acronym DOPES (Table 9.1).

Table 9.1 Possible airway and breathing complications following tracheal intubation

D	Displacement of tracheal tube (e.g. oesophagus/right main stem bronchus)
O	Obstruction of artificial airway (accumulated secretions/kinking)
P	Pneumothorax (from excessive BMV pressure/rib fractures)
E	Equipment failure (e.g. disconnected oxygen supply)
S	Stomach distension (following expired air or bag-mask ventilation)

Monitoring of the vital signs, blood gases and SpO_2 is mandatory post-resuscitation.

SpO_2 should be monitored continuously with a pulse oximeter. Although 100% oxygen is used for resuscitation, prolonged administration of high oxygen concentrations can result in pulmonary and cerebral toxicity. Once the child is stable, inspired oxygen should be gradually reduced to achieve an SpO_2 of between 94-98%.

End-tidal CO_2 ($ETCO_2$) monitoring is advisable. This will not only confirm correct initial placement of a tracheal tube but also allow continuous CO_2 monitoring during transport. A chest x-ray should be obtained to identify lung pathology, check for rib fractures, confirm the correct tracheal tube position and gastric tube position as appropriate (Figure 9.1).

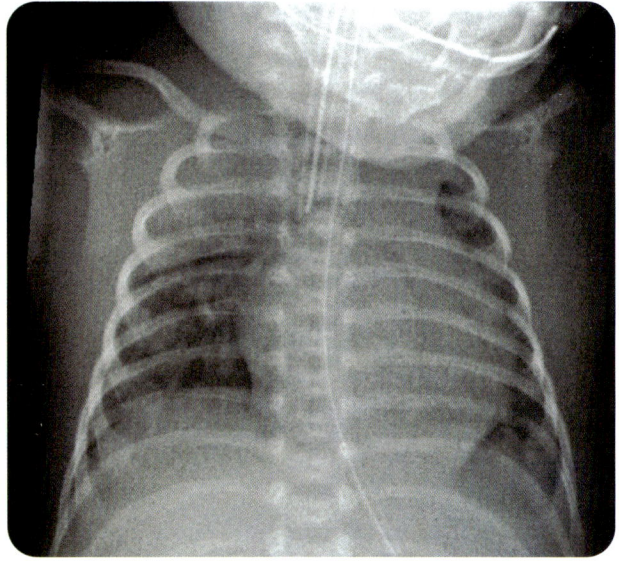

Figure 9.1 Chest x-ray showing tracheal tube at low position, causing right upper lobe collapse- this resolves when the tube is gently pulled back up the trachea.

If a resuscitated child has a tracheal tube in place and starts to make respiratory effort but remains unconscious, it is usually preferable to leave them intubated and ventilated (with appropriate sedation and analgesia) until after transfer and admission to PICU, since they can deteriorate rapidly, and reintubation during transfer is extremely hazardous.

Circulation

The aim of circulatory management is to ensure adequate organ perfusion and tissue oxygenation.

Haemodynamic function and cardiac rhythm are likely to be unstable in the immediate post-resuscitation phase. In addition to continuous ECG, SpO_2, $ETCO_2$ and BP monitoring, vital organ perfusion should be assessed by recording urine output and peripheral perfusion (CRT and skin temperature) as a minimum. Ideally, CRT should be < 2 seconds and the heart rate, blood pressure and respiratory rate should all be maintained within the age-appropriate range. Systolic BP is an indirect measure of organ perfusion and can be obtained either non-invasively or continuously via an arterial line, (particularly useful for ventilated patients). Urine output should be > 1ml kg^{-1} h^{-1} in children. Assessment of central venous pressure (CVP), a measure of preload (i.e. the filling volume of the heart) may also be appropriate in some children but will require placement of a central line. After fluid resuscitation palpation of the liver edge may also give an indication of fluid status (particularly in infants) and should normally be < 1cm beyond the costal margin.

Assessment of the child's fluid balance and circulating volume must be considered. Resuscitation boluses of isotonic saline solutions, such as 0.9% saline or Hartmann's solution may be required to optimise circulating volume. Crystalloids can be safely used peri-resuscitation but some patients may require blood or other colloids.

Maintenance fluids should be based on biochemistry evaluations and blood glucose should be measured. Glucose should be administered judiciously as required to avoid hypoglycaemia or hyperglycaemia as both conditions can have a deleterious effect on neurological outcome in critically unwell children. Careful monitoring is required. During the immediate post-resuscitation period, decisions about securing longer-term vascular access will be required (e.g. insertion of central venous cannulae to replace intraosseous access or additional lines to deliver specific medications).

Ongoing resuscitation of the child may necessitate inotrope infusions. These are preferably administered via dedicated central venous catheters. Having a central line with multiple lumens ensures that inotropes are not interrupted to deliver other medications and fluids, and avoids incompatibilities.

Commonly used inotropes include dopamine, milrinone, adrenaline and noradrenaline but consensus guidelines for specific conditions should be followed e.g. sepsis guidelines for children.

Disability and Exposure

The brain is highly vulnerable to hypoxia and ischaemia. It can be injured by direct trauma, infection, hyper/hypoglycaemia, hypocapnia, seizures or raised intracranial pressure. Secondary brain injury can be minimised by stabilising systemic blood pressure, treating seizures, normalising blood gases (taking particular care to avoid hypoxia) and correcting glucose and electrolyte abnormalities.

An assessment of neurological status should be performed early to obtain a post-resuscitation baseline, help identify neurological deficits and possibly help to predict prognosis.

The conscious level should be assessed with either the AVPU or Glasgow coma scoring system. Pupil reactivity, posturing and focal signs should also be noted and regularly recorded.

Exposure and a full examination to detect any lesions (e.g. rashes, wounds) should be undertaken and may help in making the diagnosis, informing specific management of the child. Care should be taken to respect the child's dignity and excessive hypothermia avoided especially in infants.

Other Organs

Renal function should be monitored by measuring urine output, and the serum urea and creatinine levels. Placement of a urinary catheter may be necessary. Treatment is directed towards maintaining an adequate circulating volume, which sustains renal perfusion. Hence diuretics are only indicated if decreased urine output persists after adequate fluid resuscitation. The gastrointestinal mucosa and liver can also be affected by hypoxia and ischaemia. Gastrointestinal mucosal injury can contribute to multi-organ failure, due to leakage of toxins and bacteria into the circulation. Treatment is aimed at maintaining adequate circulating volume and gut perfusion.

Further assessment

History

A comprehensive history is important to determine the cause of cardiorespiratory arrest, and plan ongoing management. This should include details about previous health/disease and medications, as well as precipitating events. Details about the initial management of the current event (e.g. delay in starting resuscitation) should also be sought, as these may influence ongoing management.

Investigations

The child's physiological parameters are likely to be deranged in the immediate post-resuscitation period; urgent haematological, biochemical, radiological and cardiological investigations may all be indicated (Table 9.2).

Optimising brain function

Cerebral perfusion

Immediately following ROSC, there may be a period of unstable cerebral blood flow. Cerebral perfusion is dependent on mean arterial pressure – hypotension or severe hypertension will compromise cerebral blood flow and may worsen any neurological injury. The aim is therefore to maintain the mean arterial pressure at, or slightly above, the child's normal level.

Seizure control

The occurrence of seizures post-resuscitation is not uncommon and an isolated event does not appear to affect outcome. However, status epilepticus is associated with a poor outcome, and therefore control of seizure activity is essential to prevent increased cerebral metabolism and potential neurological injury. Commonly used treatments for seizure (e.g. benzodiazepines, phenytoin) can cause hypotension, and the BP and ECG needs to be closely monitored.

Temperature control

Therapeutic hypothermia

Hypothermia is common following cardiorespiratory resuscitation, but there is current interest in determining if therapeutic hypothermia may help to produce optimal neuological outcome. Central hypothermia (32-34°C) may be beneficial, having been shown to improve adult neurological outcomes after VF arrests. It has an acceptable safety profile in adults and neonates, and is used in the management of newborns with hypoxic ischaemic encephalopathy.

There is limited information about its efficacy in older children with cardiorespiratory arrest. At the time of writing, there are

Table 9.2: Post-resuscitation investigations

Investigation	Rationale
Arterial blood gas (plus lactate)	• Ensure adequate ventilation • Assess tissue perfusion
Biochemistry	• Assess renal function • Maintain normoglycaemia • Assess electrolyte balance (especially Na^+, K^+, Mg^{2+}, Ca^+) • Liver function tests to look for ischaemic injury
Full blood count Clotting screen Group and Save	• Assess haemoglobin level and exclude anaemia • Monitor infection markers e.g. white cell count, CRP etc • Identify underlying blood disorders • Assess any coagulopathy from sepsis or ischaemia • Allows for urgent crossmatch
Chest x-ray	• Establish position of tracheal tube, central venous lines, gastric tube (as appropriate) • Detect underlying pathology (primary respiratory or cardiac disease, aspiration) • Exclude pneumothorax/rib fractures • Establish heart size

Other investigations as indicated (e.g. head CT or pelvis x-rays, cardiac echography, 12-lead ECG, serum and urine toxicology)

several studies, exploring the use of therapeutic hypothermia on this group of patients.

The current consensus for carrying out therapeutic hypothermia is as follows:

1. A child who regains a spontaneous circulation, but remains comatose after cardiorespiratory arrest, is cooled to a core temperature of 32-34°C for at least 24 h.

2. The successfully resuscitated child with hypothermia and return of spontaneous circulation should not be rewarmed actively unless the core temperature is below 32°C. Following a period of mild hypothermia, the child is rewarmed slowly at 0.25-0.5°C h^{-1}.

3. Complications of mild therapeutic hypothermia include increased risk of infection, cardiovascular instability, coagulopathy, hyperglycaemia, and electrolyte

abnormalities such as hypophosphataemia and hypomagnesaemia.

Hyperthermia (hyperpyrexia)

Within the first 48 hours post-resuscitation, hyperthermia is common. There appears to be a correlation between hyperthermia and poor neurological outcome (i.e. the higher the fever, the poorer the outcome). For this reason, fever should be aggressively managed with antipyretic medications and/or active cooling.

Blood glucose control

Normalisation of blood glucose levels is important as both hypoglycaemia and hyperglycaemia have potential negative effects on outcome. Nevertheless aggressive glucose control can be associated with inadvertent profound hypoglycaemia and frequent blood glucose estimations must be performed with interventions initiated, according to local policies. There is currently a multi-centre trial to evaluate tight glucose control for critically ill children in the UK.

Analgesia and sedation

Early treatment of pain and the maintenance of an adequate level of sedation are priorities in the care of the child.

- Do not use a muscle relaxant without sedation and analgesia

- An intubated child should not be agitated as ventilation will be ineffective and transport will be hazardous. Always give adequate sedation and analgesia

- Ensure adequate analgesia not just sedation. Know the properties of the drugs administered and be aware that most cause hypotension, anticipate the side effects.

- Sedation may not be necessary in profound coma and may interfere with neurological evaluation; always discuss such cases with the local PICU for guidance.

Facilitating safe patient transfer

Following stabilisation, the child should be safely transferred to an appropriate PICU facility for definitive care. The decision to transfer should be made only after discussion between senior members of the PICU team, the clinical emergency team leader and the child's primary team (if available for consultation). Other considerations pre-transfer are listed in Figure 9.2.

The transfer team must be skilled and experienced personnel, able to continue optimal clinical observation and perform all emergency interventions that may be necessary to manage a critically ill child. In the UK, a dedicated paediatric transfer team will usually be involved. There are some circumstances however, (such as intra-cranial bleeds requiring urgent surgical evacuation) where rapid transfer by the most experienced available local team members will be in the child's best interest.

Care of the rescuers/debriefing

It is important that all resuscitation events are audited (including the National Cardiac Arrest audit). Whether the

- Stabilise the child (ongoing or recurrent cardiorespiratory arrest precludes transfer)
- Arrange the most appropriate mode of transport
- Check all equipment and medications, particularly oxygen supplies, immediately prior to transfer
- Ensure a secure airway (aspirate secretions before transfer)
- Confirm secure and patent circulatory access (usually 2 functioning cannulae)
- Transfer all medication/fluid infusions and monitoring to portable transport devices
- Deflate stomach with passage of a gastric tube
- Contact PICU to update them of child's clinical status and provide estimated time of arrival before departure
- Prepare full and clear records of the event including all interventions (copies of notes, drug charts, X-rays is ideal)
- Inform child's parents of transfer details and ensure they have appropriate means of transport to the PICU

Figure 9.2 Pre-transfer considerations

resuscitation attempt was successful or not, healthcare providers should be supported and given constructive feedback on performance (Chapter 14).

The relatives of the child will require considerable ongoing support in the event of both successful and unsuccessful resuscitation attempts. The early involvement of pastoral/counselling services should be considered.

Key learning points

▸ ROSC following cardiopulmonary resuscitation is merely the first step in the continuous process of resuscitation management

▸ The ongoing management of seriously ill children includes appropriate vital sign monitoring, supportive therapies based on continuous ABCDE assessment and safe transfer to a PICU facility

▸ The prognosis for children following cardiorespiratory arrest depends on many factors, including the quality of post-resuscitation care

▸ The ability to predict the neurological outcome of children following cardioplumonary resuscitation remains limited

Further reading

Brierley J, Carcillo JA, Choong K et al. Clinical practice parameters for hemodynamic support of pediatric and neonatal septic shock: 2007 update from the American College of Critical Care Medicine. Critical Care Medicine 2009 37(2):666-88.

Special Situations in Paediatric Resuscitation

CHAPTER 10

Learning outcomes

To understand:
- How airway and breathing are changed in special situations
- How circulation may be compromised in anaphylaxis or dehydration
- The common electrolyte abnormalities following ABCDE principles

In childhood, cardiorespiratory arrest is mainly secondary to illness and the usual outcome is poor; therefore, strategies to recognise and manage the primary condition may prevent decompensated respiratory or circulatory failure.

Respiratory and/or circulatory failure are the first steps of this pathway and their management does not require a precise diagnosis, as it is based on the ABCDE approach. However, in certain circumstances, the knowledge of the underlying disease may help to determine specific management and improve the child's outcome.

Laryngotracheitis (croup)

Croup is defined as an acute clinical syndrome of inspiratory stridor, barking cough, hoarseness, and variable degrees of respiratory distress. Acute viral laryngotracheobronchitis (viral croup) is the most common form of croup and accounts for over 95% of laryngeotracheal infections.

Parainfluenza viruses are the most common pathogens but other respiratory viruses (e.g. respiratory syncytial virus [RSV] and adenoviruses) produce a similar clinical picture.

The majority of children with croup are managed at home, whilst those in mild to moderate respiratory distress may need admission and supportive treatment.

Steroids are used to reduce laryngeal oedema. A few children may require intubation owing to a combination of exhaustion and respiratory failure.

Airway – This is at risk of marked swelling of the larynx and trachea which can lead to partial or complete obstruction of the airway, if the oedema progresses.

Breathing – Respiratory rate and work of breathing increase with progressive airway obstruction.

Circulation – This is normal until decompensated respiratory failure develops.

Disability – Exhaustion is an ominous sign, indicating decompensated respiratory failure.

Exposure – This will show how hard the child is working, by seeing the use of accessory muscles.

Management of decompensation

1. Open the airway if required with head tilt chin lift or jaw thrust.

2. Give 100% oxygen and start bag-mask ventilation (BMV) if required.

Intubation may be a challenge. Help from an experienced team member, anaesthetist, or ENT surgeon capable of performing a tracheotomy should be requested.

A narrower tracheal tube than would normally be expected may be required.

Respiratory failure is due to upper airway obstruction and will improve when the airway is adequately managed.

Epiglottitis

This is an intense swelling of the epiglottis and surrounding tissues caused almost exclusively by Haemophilus influenzae type B. It is predominantly seen in children aged 1-6 years. It is now uncommon owing to Hib vaccination in UK children.

Typically, the child suddenly develops a high fever and is lethargic, pale and toxic. He is usually sitting immobile with his mouth open and chin raised. There may be excessive drooling owing to an inability to swallow saliva as it is painful to do so.

Airway – Swelling of the epiglottis leads to severe obstruction of the upper airway. Complete obstruction is fatal and can occur if the condition is untreated or if the child becomes distressed (e.g. by attempting to examine his throat, forcing him to lie down or performing other frightening manoeuvres such as inserting an intravenous cannula or taking a lateral X-ray of the neck).

Breathing – There is an increased respiratory rate and effort, a muffled or hoarse voice, soft respiratory stridor and absent or minimal cough. Respiratory failure is due to the upper airway obstruction.

Circulation – This is normal until decompensated respiratory failure develops. Inappropriate management can lead to sudden cardiorespiratory arrest because of complete airway obstruction.

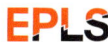

Disability – Tiredness and decreasing level of consciousness are worrying signs of decompensated respiratory failure. Exhaustion is a pre-terminal state.

Exposure – The child may be dribbling saliva, looking flushed, 'toxic' and unwell. There is no specific rash to see.

Management

The child should be left with parents, and under close observation, while arrangements are made for an experienced team to secure his airway by tracheal intubation under controlled conditions.

Once the airway has been secured, normalisation of breathing is the rule. Thereafter, with intravenous antibiotics, the prognosis is excellent as the underlying infection usually responds quickly to treatment.

If cardiorespiratory arrest occurs, the child should be ventilated by BMV (with pressure limiting valve being overridden if necessary) and this should be continued until the child is intubated or a surgical airway obtained.

Bronchiolitis

Bronchiolitis is a common, serious respiratory infection of infancy caused by RSV in 75% of cases; the remainder are due to parainfluenza, influenza and adenoviruses. It occurs mainly in the winter and is the reason for 1-2% of all infant admissions to hospital. Ninety per cent of patients are aged 1-9 months and it is uncommon after 1 year. As there is no specific treatment for bronchiolitis, its management is supportive.

Airway – Nasal obstruction from secretions can occur.

Breathing – The inflammatory process causes oedema of the small airways and copious secretions, which can lead to hypoxia and hypercapnia; a ventilation-perfusion mismatch occurs. Apnoea and exhaustion can also occur.

Circulation – This is normal until decompensated respiratory failure occurs.

Disability – As with the previous respiratory disorders, tiredness, confusion and agitation reflect failing respiratory compensation. Decreasing level of consciousness is an ominous sign and exhaustion is a preteminal event.

Exposure – The child will shows signs of increased respiratory effort but there is no specific rash associated with this condition. The use of respiratory muscles with head bobbing and nasal flaring may be present (as would be determined in the B section of the assessment).

Management

Gentle suction of the nose will remove secretions if nasal obstruction impairs air entry.

The ventilation-perfusion mismatch may necessitate mechanical ventilation, although many children may be managed by continuous positive airway pressure (CPAP) through a well-fitted interface (nasal prongs or facial masks). Non-invasive ventilation is the first choice of management for respiratory failure in infants with bronchiolitis in many centres.

Mechanical ventilation is required in < 2% of infants admitted to hospital. This may be due to recurrent apnoea, exhaustion or hypercapnia and hypoxia owing to small airway obstruction.

Coma

The child's conscious level may be altered by illness, injury or intoxication. The level of awareness decreases from alert (A) to stages of drowsiness (mild reduction in alertness and increase in hours of sleep) but responsive to voice (V), to responsive only to pain (P), and finally to unconsciousness (U) (unrousable/unresponsive). Levels of consciousness can be remembered by the acronym AVPU.

Airway – As the child's level of consciousness diminishes, the likelihood of obstruction of the airway increases owing to the loss of tone of soft tissue. When the child becomes reactive only to pain, there maybe loss of protective cough and gag reflex, hence aspiration of stomach contents may occur.

Breathing – Coma may lead to slow respiratory rate and/or inadequate respiratory effort.

Circulation – According to the cause of the coma, circulation can be affected (e.g. hypovolaemic shock in diabetic ketoacidosis, septic shock, hypovolaemic shock in trauma) and should be managed accordingly.

Disability – The assessment is based on AVPU, posture and pupil reaction. Recording these values is essential and form part of the ongoing assessment and management of the child. After the initial assessment of ABCDE with interventions being carried out, more detailed neurological assessment is required to determine the cause of the change in the level of consciousness.

Exposure – Causes such as meningococcaemia or other infective causes, vasculitis, SLE etc. may cause a decreased conscious level. The associated dermal manifestations can help make the diagnosis.

Management

Open the airway and maintain its patency by appropriate means (e.g. airway opening manoeuvres, nasopharyngeal or oropharyngeal airway adjuncts, or tracheal intubation may be required).

If protection against aspiration is required because of loss of the protective upper airway reflexes, intubation must be performed by rapid sequence induction of anaesthesia to avoid an increase in intracranial pressure (Chapter 4). Ventilatory support will then be required.

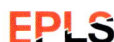

Seizures

The neurological status should be assessed and treated only after airway, breathing and circulation have been assessed and managed.

Airway – This is at risk of becoming or can be obstructed during a fit. This may be due to secretions or tongue/soft tissue hypotonia, with loss of the protective upper airway reflexes.

Breathing – Respiratory failure is due to airway obstruction or a decreased level of consciousness slowing the respiratory rate. Respiratory arrest can occur due to central nervous system depression; this is more likely if the child is receiving antiepileptic drugs (e.g. benzodiazepines) in the emergency treatment of seizures because they have respiratory depressant side effects.

Circulation – This is generally normal until decompensated respiratory failure. However, if the aetiology of the seizure is associated with other diseases (e.g. meningococcal disease or head trauma), circulatory failure may present earlier.

Disability – Seizures should be controlled by antiepileptic drugs according to national protocols. The first-line therapy is a benzodiazepine (diazepam or lorazepam). The blood glucose level should always be measured as hypoglycaemia is a treatable cause.

Exposure – As with coma, the skin may reveal the cause for the seizure such as infective causes, neurocutaneous disorders or other disorders, and help specialists in determining further management.

Management

Open the airway and maintain patency by appropriate means.

If the child remains hypoxic after airway opening, BMV with oxygen should be performed. Tracheal intubation and ventilation may sometimes be necessary to protect the airway and prevent aspiration of stomach contents.

Anaphylaxis

Anaphylaxis is a rare but life-threatening generalised or systemic hypersensitivity reaction involving several systems. The most common causes are medications (e.g. antibiotics, aspirin, non-steroidal anti-inflammatory drugs), latex, stinging insects (e.g. wasps, bees) and food (e.g. seafood, peanuts). Anaphylaxis should be considered when two or more systems are affected, predominant ones being involved include cutaneous, respiratory, cardiovascular, neurological or gastrointestinal systems.

Airway – This is at risk of becoming obstructed. The child may have a stridor and signs of respiratory failure due to laryngeal oedema and soft-tissue swelling.

Breathing – Respiratory failure may also be due to bronchospasm.

Circulation – Vasodilation causes relative hypovolaemia and increased capillary permeability with extravasation of intravascular fluids into surrounding tissues.

Disability – Decompensated circulatory +/or respiratory failure can lead to a decreasing level of consciousness and is a worrying sign.

Exposure – Flushing, pallor, urticaria.

Management (Figure 10.1)

1. Remove the likely allergen (e.g. antibiotics, blood transfusion).

2. Open airway.

3. Give 100% oxygen with BMV if required. Consider early intubation, particularly in children with lingual, labial and oropharyngeal swelling, and with hoarseness. Early involvement of an experienced anaesthetist is mandatory, as it may be a progressive condition, hence airway management before its total obstruction is an absolute must.

4. Give adrenaline intramuscularly to all children with signs of airway swelling, breathing difficulty or circulatory failure (Table 10.1). Repeat adrenaline in 5 minutes if no clinical improvement.

Table 10.1 IM adrenaline dosages for anaphylaxis

Age	Dose (1:1000 solution)
< 6 yrs	150 mcg (0.15ml)
6-12 yrs	300 mcg (0.3ml)
> 12 yrs	500 mcg (0.5ml)

5. If the child's clinical manifestations do not respond to medications give 20 ml kg^{-1} IV crystalloid (Chapter 6).

6. Give antihistamine (chlorphenamine):

< 6 months	250 mcg kg^{-1} IM or slow IV
6 months-6 years	2.5 mg IM or slow IV
6-12 years	5 mg IM or slow IV
> 12 years	10 mg IM or slow IV

7. For severe or recurrent reactions and patients with asthma, give hydrocortisone:

< 6 months	25 mg IM or slow IV
6 months-6 years	50 mg IM or slow IV
6-12 years	100 mg IM or slow IV
> 12 years	200 mg IM or slow IV

Chapter 10 Special Situations in Paediatric Resuscitation

Anaphylaxis algorithm

Anaphylactic reaction?

↓

Airway, **B**reathing, **C**irculation, **D**isability, **E**xposure

↓

Diagnosis - look for:
- Acute onset of illness
- Life-threatening Airway and/or Breathing and/or Circulation problems [1]
- And usually skin changes

↓

- **Call for help**
- Lie patient flat
- Raise patient's legs

↓

Adrenaline [2]

↓

When skills and equipment available:
- Establish airway
- High flow oxygen
- IV fluid challenge [3]
- Chlorphenamine [4]
- Hydrocortisone [5]

Monitor:
- Pulse oximetry
- ECG
- Blood pressure

---

[1] Life-threatening problems:
- **Airway:** swelling, hoarseness, stridor
- **Breathing:** rapid breathing, wheeze, fatigue, cyanosis, SpO_2 < 92%, confusion
- **Circulation:** pale, clammy, low blood pressure, faintness, drowsy/coma

---

[2] Adrenaline *(give IM unless experienced with IV adrenaline)*
IM doses of 1:1000 adrenaline (repeat after 5 min if no better)
- Adult: 500 micrograms IM (0.5 mL)
- Child more than 12 years: 500 micrograms IM (0.5 mL)
- Child 6 -12 years: 300 micrograms IM (0.3 mL)
- Child less than 6 years: 150 micrograms IM (0.15 mL)

Adrenaline IV to be given **only by experienced specialists**
Titrate: Adults 50 micrograms; Children 1 microgram/kg

[3] IV fluid challenge:
Adult - 500 – 1000 mL
Child - crystalloid 20 mL/kg

Stop IV colloid if this might be the cause of anaphylaxis

---

	[4] Chlorphenamine (IM or slow IV)	**[5] Hydrocortisone** (IM or slow IV)
Adult or child more than 12 years	10 mg	200 mg
Child 6 - 12 years	5 mg	100 mg
Child 6 months to 6 years	2.5 mg	50 mg
Child less than 6 months	250 micrograms/kg	25 mg

March 2008

Figure 10.1 Anaphylaxis algorithm

Dehydration

Dehydration arises from increased fluid loss and/or decreased intake which cannot be corrected by the kidneys. Hypovolaemic shock ensues when there is loss of central circulatory homeostatic mechanisms. The major causes of dehydration in children are burns, trauma, gastrointestinal disorders and diabetic ketoacidosis. Signs of dehydration often precede those of circulatory failure.

Moderate and severe dehydration require accurate replacement of fluid deficit with monitoring of plasma electrolyte levels. In diabetic ketoacidosis, fluid replacement should be cautious after the initial resuscitation as fluid overload and cerebral oedema may occur.

Airway – This is safe if consciousness is not compromised.

Breathing – Respiratory rate increases to compensate for the acidosis due to dehydration, diabetic ketoacidosis or other forms of shock.

Circulation – Assess for signs of circulatory failure.

Disability – The child's conscious level decrease as his cerebral perfusion diminishes. This worsens as he becomes more hypovolaemic; this can lead to the child can become obtunded.

Exposure – Skin turgour, any associated rashes, the presence of burns (assessing the extent and depth of burn) or any trauma should be noted.

Management

1. Open airway.
2. Give 100% oxygen and BMV if required.
3. Obtain vascular access and give boluses of fluid ($20\ ml\ kg^{-1}$) as indicated by regular assessment.

Respiratory distress in a child with a tracheostomy

This may be caused by obstruction of the tracheostomy tube leading to ineffective ventilation. The tube should be cleared or removed and replaced; if a clean tube is not available then ventilation at the tracheostomy stoma site should be given until the tube is cleaned. If the child's upper airway is patent, it may be possible to provide BMV via the mouth and nose using a conventional bag and mask while the tracheal stoma site is occluded.

Children in intensive care

Critically ill children are at high risk of cardiorespiratory arrest owing to their illness or treatment (e.g. postoperative complications following cardiac surgery). At greatest risk are children who have had a previous cardiorespiratory arrest.

Electrolyte abnormalities

Some electrolyte disturbances can cause cardiac arrhythmias, cardiorespiratory arrest or can make resuscitation less effective.

In some circumstances the correction of an anticipated electrolyte disturbance may be started, based on clinical parameters, before laboratory results are available.

Potassium (K^+)

The causes of hyperkalaemia and hypokalaemia are given in Table 10.2.

Table 10.2 Causes of potassium disturbance

Hyperkalaemia	Hypokalaemia
Renal failure (acute/chronic)	Gastrointestinal losses e.g. diarrhoea, vomiting
Acidosis	Alkalosis
Adrenal insufficiency • Addison's disease • Secondary	
Excessive potassium intake	Volume depletion
Intake of K^+ sparing medication	Diuretics
Cell lysis e.g. in tumour treatment, tissue infarction	Insufficient potassium intake
Haemolysis	Malnutrition
Massive blood transfusions	Insufficient K^+ intake

The K^+ gradient, from the intracellular to extracellular space, determines the conduction of the myocardial cells and therefore their contractility. Even limited increases in serum K^+ can be responsible for decreased conduction and diminished cardiac contractility. Arterial pH has a direct effect on K^+; acidosis increases serum K^+ (by 0.5-1.1 mmol l^{-1} for each 0.1 decrease in pH).

Hyperkalaemia

Hyperkalaemia ($K^+ > 7$ mmol l^{-1}) is characterised by muscular weakness, paralytic ileus, respiratory arrest and heart conduction disturbances leading to arrhythmias and eventually to cardiac arrest.

Typical ECG changes seen in hyperkalaemia are dependent on both the K^+ level and the associated rate of increase in K^+ level.

Initially there is T wave elevation but this progresses into an idioventricular rhythm and ventricular fibrillation as serum K^+ rises.

False hyperkalaemia values can result from haemolysis of the blood due to difficult capillary blood sampling.

Management

The treatment of hyperkalaemia is dependent on the speed of occurrence of the symptoms and the clinical state of the child, or if they show toxic ECG changes. It includes:

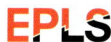

1. Intravenous calcium chloride given as a bolus, or over 2-5 minutes if the child is not in cardiorespiratory arrest to antagonise the toxic effects of hyperkalaemia at the myocardial cell membrane.
2. Sodium bicarbonate (if acidosis or renal failure is present).
3. Insulin-glucose infusion.
4. Salbutamol administration either via a nebuliser or intravenously.
5. Haemodialysis/peritoneal dialysis.

If the child shows elevation of the serum K^+ levels only with no symptoms, excess K^+ may be removed from the body by the use of:

1. Diuretics: furosemide.
2. Ion exchange resins (calcium resonium given orally or rectally). Onset of the effect is slow but this treatment can be started early (as soon as the K^+ level is increased).

Hypokalaemia

Hypokalaemia ($K^+ < 3.5$ mmol l^{-1}) is characterised by muscular weakness, constipation, paresthesia and tetany.

Severe hypokalaemia (< 2.5 mmol l^{-1}) can cause life-threatening arrhythmias (VF, VT, PEA or asystole), paralysis, rhabdomyolysis, paralytic ileus and metabolic alkalosis.

Management

Treatment of hypokalaemia (2.5 - 3.5 mmol l^{-1}) includes the early recognition of the cause. Patients treated with digitalis are at special risk of developing arrhythmias.

Treatment of severe hypokalaemia (< 2.5 mmol l^{-1}) or hypokalaemia associated with arrhythmias consists of careful intravenous K^+ infusion (preferably via central access) under ECG monitoring.

This is best performed in a PICU or on a high-dependency unit as there is a high risk of cardiorespiratory arrest from arrhythmia. An infusion of 0.5 mmol kg^{-1} h^{-1} of KCl is given until the arrhythmia resolves and/or the K^+ level is > 3.5 mmol l^{-1}. A total dose of 2-3 mmol kg^{-1} KCl may be required; administration of K^+ should be reduced as soon as the child is clinically stable.

Calcium

Hypercalcaemia

Hypercalcaemia usually presents as long-standing anorexia, malaise, weight loss, failure to thrive and vomiting. Other symptoms are convulsions, coma, polyuria, dehydration, hypokalaemia, bradycardia, arterial hypertension and ECG changes (e.g., short QT, widening of QRS complexes, AV block).

Causes include:

- Hyperparathyroidism
- Hypervitaminosis D or A
- Idiopathic hypercalcaemia of infancy
- Malignancy
- Thiazide diuretic abuse
- Skeletal disorders

Management

Treatment of hypercalcaemia is mandatory when symptoms appear.

Initial treatment consists of fluid resuscitation with 0.9% saline. Infusion of twice the calculated basic requirement is delivered, providing the degree of dehydration, cardiac function and blood pressure permit significant fluid administration. Levels of both serum K^+ and magnesium (Mg^{2+}) should be monitored. Furosemide can be useful in patients with fluid overload; however, in children with renal insufficiency and oliguria, dialysis is necessary.

Hypocalcaemia

Causes include:

- Hypoparathyroidism (di George syndrome, magnesium deficiency, familial)
- Vitamin D deficiency
- Vitamin D resistance
- Hypoproteinaemia
- Phosphate intoxication

Specific symptoms are:

- Signs of neuronal irritation
- Convulsions
- Laryngeal stridor
- Rickets
- ECG changes: QT prolongation, AV block, ventricular fibrillation

Non-specific symptoms are vomiting, muscular weakness and irritability.

Management

The treatment of severe hypocalcaemia (without hypomagnesaemia) includes intravenous or intraosseous administration of calcium gluconate. Oral supplements of calcium may be needed.

If hypocalcaemia is associated with hypomagnaesemia, Mg^{2+} replacement will also be necessary.

Diabetic Ketoacidosis

Diabetic ketoacidosis (DKA) is caused by low insulin levels and associated increase in other hormones such as glucagon, cortisol and growth hormone. This results in the following key features of DKA:

Hyperglycaemia (blood glucose> 11 mmol l^{-1})

Hypersomolality

Ketonaemia

Metabolic acidosis (pH< 7.3, bicarbonate< 15 mmol l^{-1})

Clinical features include dehydration, abnormal deep sighing respiration (Kussmaul breaths), vomiting and drowsiness. The clinical history may include increased urine output, increased thirst, weight loss, abdominal pain and confusion.

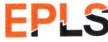

It is important not to overestimate the degree of dehydration. A guide is outlined in Table 10.3.

Table 10.3 Dehydration Guide

Mild (3%) dehydration	Moderate (5%) dehydration	Severe (8%) dehydration
Only just clinically detectable	Dry mucous membranes Reduced skin turgour	Additionally sunken eyes, poor capillary return

DKA can be fatal. Cerebral oedema accounts for 57-87% of all DKA deaths. Other causes include aspiration pneumonia and hypokalaemia. Because of this it is important to **recognise DKA early and get senior help.** The aim is to rehydrate but minimise the risk of cerebral oedema.

Airway – This is safe if consciousness is not compromised.

Breathing – Children are often breathing quickly to compensate for their metabolic acidosis.

Circulation – Assess for signs of circulatory failure. Signs of shock include poor peripheral pulses, poor capillary refill time and hypotension. Assess the degree of dehydration.

Disability – Assess level of consciousness using GCS or AVPU. Continue hourly neurological observations. Monitor blood glucose, sodium and potassium.

Exposure – Fever is not a feature of DKA. If present, take blood cultures and consider antibiotics.

Management

1. Ensure the airway is patent.
2. Intubation should be avoided unless the patient has a GCS< 8, has a respiratory arrest or has poor respiratory effort. Insert a nasogastric tube to prevent aspiration of vomit.
3. Obtain vascular access and check blood gases, blood sugar, and serum potassium. Attach a cardiac monitor. If shocked (see above) give 10ml kg^{-1} of 0.9% saline. These boluses can be repeated up to a maximum of 30ml kg^{-1}.
4. Avoid using bicarbonate as its use is associated with an increased risk of cerebral oedema.
5. Commence fluids with 0.9% saline with potassium as per your unit protocol (British Society for Paediatric Endocrinology and Diabetes (BSPED) guidelines).
6. If there are any signs of reduced conscious level or raised intracranial pressure assume that the patient has cerebral oedema. **Get senior help immediately.**
7. Start insulin infusion approximately 1 hour after maintenance and replacement fluids started, as per protocol, at 0.05 to 0.1 units kg^{-1} hour^{-1}.

Children with cardiac problems

Cardiac problems are relatively common (6-8 per 1000 live births) and may present throughout childhood, although most commonly in the neonatal period. Clinical features include the presence of a murmur plus or minus cyanosis. There may also be signs of cardiac failure, such as tachypneoa, crackles on lung auscultation and hepatomegaly and/or poor systemic perfusion such as prolonged capillary refill time, poor or absent pulses and hypotension.

Cardiac problems can be classified as:

1. Congenital cardiac problems including cyanotic (e.g. transposition of great arteries); obstructive (e.g. coarctation of aorta) and hypoplastic (e.g. hypoplastic left heart) lesions. When these babies present unexpectedly in the neonatal period, a prostaglandin infusion such as dinoprostone, PGE2, is usually required to open the ductus arteriosus. Other congenital cardiac lesions include septal defects (e.g. ventricular septal defects, (VSD)) which are generally less severe, present later and do not require prostaglandin. VSDs are the most common form of congenital heart disease 25-30% and the infants usually present in cardiac failure with signs including tachypnoea, tachycardia, poor perfusion, pallor, hepatomegaly, and crackles in the lung bases and additionally with failure to thrive.

2. Later onset, acquired problems (e.g. myocarditis, cardiomyopathy), usually present with features of cardiac failure with signs including tachycardia, tachypnoea and hepatomegaly.

3. Rhythm disturbance (Chapter 7).

Airway – This is safe if consciousness is not compromised.

Breathing – Several key clinical features include tachypneoa (cardiac failure) and low saturations (particularly cyanotic congenital lesions). A cyanotic congenital cardiac problem is suspected if there is no improvement in saturations when oxygen is administered. In older children with an established cardiac diagnosis, it is helpful to establish and target usual oxygen saturations for them. In heart failure there may be crepitations at the lung bases on auscultation.

Circulation – There may be signs of circulatory compromise or even shock, such as tachycardia, poor peripheral pulses, prolonged capillary refill time and possible hypotension. Other problems such as poor feeding or sepsis may lead to hypovolaemia and fluid boluses may be required but these should be given with caution (see management). An infusion of prostaglandin should be commenced if a neonate is suspected of having a congenital cardiac problem.

Disability – An abnormal conscious level may reflect impaired end-organ function due to respiratory or circulatory compromise. Hypoglycaemia is more likely in a sick infant. Monitor electrolytes particularly if the child is receiving diuretics or drugs to manage cardiac failure.

Exposure – Skin perfusion should be assessed. Although fever may be related to prostaglandin infusion, consider the possibility of sepsis if fever is present.

Management

1. Get senior help immediately.
2. Give high-flow oxygen especially when the diagnosis is uncertain. A brief period of oxygen is unlikely to close a patent ductus arteriosus. Discuss with a paediatric cardiologist as soon as possible.

3. Commence a prostaglandin infusion when a neonatal duct dependent problem is suspected e.g. in cases of sudden unexplained deterioration in the first week or so after birth. Duct dependent lesions may be due to congenital cyanotic, obstructive or hypoplastic cardiac conditions. Prostaglandin infusions can be given peripherally, or via an intraosseous line, but must be on a dedicated line and should not be given by bolus. Higher doses may cause apnoea requiring respiratory support.

4. Cautious use of diuretics may be helpful in cardiac failure (e.g. VSD) and additional respiratory support may be required.

5. Consider cautious fluid resuscitation using boluses of 10 ml kg^{-1} of 0.9% NaCl up to 30 ml kg^{-1} in total. Carefully reassess after each bolus as worsening tachycardia or liver enlargement suggest fluid overload and then diuretics rather than fluid resuscitation would be indicated.

6. Consider discussing with a paediatric intensivist as more sophisticated monitoring (e.g. invasive blood pressure) and therapy (e.g. vasoactive drugs) as well as transfer to a specialist centre, may be required.

Sepsis

Sepsis is a common cause of death in children. It may be accompanied by organ dysfunction (severe sepsis) or hypotension (septic shock). Prompt recognition and management is vital.

Airway – This may be compromised by reduced level of consciousness (e.g. meningitis, any infection causing shock).

Breathing – Children may have respiratory distress (tachypnoea, increased work of breathing) or respiratory failure due to the underlying condition (pneumonia) or as a result of other processes (septic response). Ventilatory support may be required.

Circulation – Children may have tachycardia, prolonged capillary refill time, poor peripheral pulses and possibly hypotension (cold shock). Sometimes sepsis results in vasodilatation with warm peripheries and early hypotension (warm shock). Fluid maldistribution is common and severe sepsis often additionally causes myocardial dysfunction. Compensated circulatory failure may mask the true severity of the illness and urgency required in management. Careful assessment is required.

Disability – An abnormal conscious level may reflect impaired end-organ function due to respiratory or circulatory compromise. However, abnormal neurological status may reflect the underlying condition itself (e.g. meningitis). Blood glucose should always be checked as hypoglycaemia is relatively common and should be rechecked if new problems (e.g. seizures) are encountered.

Exposure – This can give clues to the diagnosis. Look for rashes (e.g. meningococcal disease, toxic shock) or other skin lesions (e.g. herpes simplex).

Management

1. Get senior help immediately.

2. Give 100% oxygen initially. Consider early intubation by an experienced anaesthetist especially if > 40 ml kg^{-1} of IV fluid has been required.

3. Administer antibiotics rapidly. The choice depends on the suspected site of infection and organism (and resistance pattern if known) – refer to local antibiotic guidelines. Third generation cephalosporins (e.g. cefotaxime) are often appropriate. Consider the possibility of other organisms (e.g. herpes simplex).

4. Fluid resuscitation using boluses of 20 ml kg^{-1} of 0.9% Sodium Chloride initially. Do not hesitate to use the intraosseous (IO) route. Large quantities of fluid may be required. Carefully reassess after each bolus.

5. Vasoactive drugs may be required. These IV infusions optimise cardiac output by improving cardiac contractility (dopamine, adrenaline), raising systemic vascular resistance (noradrenaline) or raising the heart rate (chronotropes). They should be considered in children especially where shock is unresponsive to fluid boluses. Dopamine is generally the first line inotrope in children and can be given peripherally; other vasoactives can initially be administered by the IO route until central access is secured.

6. Seek specialist advice early as more sophisticated monitoring (e.g. invasive blood pressure), management decisions (blood product use) and adjunctive treatments may be required.

> ### Key learning points
>
> - The conditions described in this chapter are common causes of cardiorespiratory arrest in children
> - Use the ABCDE approach for early recognition and treatment to prevent cardiorespiratory arrest
> - Call for expert help early when specialist procedures are needed

Further reading

ILCOR Worksheets on therapeutic hypothermia
http://www.americanheart.org/presenter.jhtml?identifier=3066827.

Resuscitation Council UK guidance on the management of anaphylaxis
http://www.resus.org.uk/pages/faqAna.htm.

www.bsped.org.uk. Under clinical endorsed guidelines. BPSED recommended DKA guidelines 2009 (updated 2013).

Dellinger RP. Surviving Sepsis Campaign: International Guidelines For Management Of Severe Sepsis And Septic Shock, 2012. Intensive Care Medicine. 2013. 39; 165-228.

Hoffman JIE, Kaplan S. The incidence of congenital heart disease. Journal of the American College of Cardiology. 2002; 12 (39). 1890-1900.

http://publications.nice.org.uk/guidance/ CG137 Appendix F: Protocols for treating convulsive status epilepticus in children 2011 (updated Dec 2013).

http://www.survivingsepsis.org. International guidelines for management of severe sepsis and septic shock CritCare Med;2013:41(2)580-637.

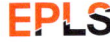

The Injured Child

CHAPTER 11

Learning outcomes

To understand:
- The AcBCDE approach in trauma
- The need for in-line cervical spine immobilisation
- The use of primary and secondary surveys
- The priorities in managing head, cervical spine, thoracic, abdominal and limb injuries
- The management of children with burns
- The management of children following drowning

Trauma is the leading cause of death and disability worldwide in children over 1 year. Blunt trauma is seen in 80% of paediatric cases in the UK; of these, two thirds of life-threatening paediatric trauma is related to brain injury.

Injury patterns in children vary from those seen in adults, owing to the different physiological and anatomical responses to trauma. In children, there is a relatively smaller muscle mass, less subcutaneous tissue and increased elasticity of ribs and other bones. This means that in the child more of the impacting energy is transmitted to underlying organs such as the lungs (often without rib fractures) or abdomen (with damage to visceral organs). Internal injury must therefore always be considered as there may have been significant force involved without external signs being present. The history of the mechanism of injury must always be sought and clinical consequences of how the impacting energy has been dispersed through the child's body must be considered.

When dealing with an injured child it is vital that appropriate resuscitative measures are carried out as soon as problems are identified. These measures must be applied in a structured manner to ensure maximal benefit. This structured approach consists of the primary survey (AcBCDE) and resuscitation followed by:

- X-ray series: chest and pelvis. Note that the cervical spine x-ray may be deferred as part of the secondary survey
- Secondary survey
- Emergency treatment
- Definitive care

The general principles of resuscitation for the injured child are similar to those of the critically ill child but there are a few important differences, described in this chapter.

Primary survey

Airway compromise, respiratory failure and circulatory failure can co-exist following trauma. The primary survey is a systematic rapid evaluation which identifies life-threatening problems using the AcBCDE approach. It is completed in the first minutes of the initial assessment of the child.

Treat first what kills first

- **Ac** **Airway and cervical spine** stabilisation
- **B** **Breathing** oxygenation and ventilation (consider tension pneumothorax)
- **C** **Circulation** and external haemorrhage control
- **D** **Disability** Neurological status (AVPU, pupils, posture)
- **E** **Exposure (and Environment)** undress the child, and understand the history and consequences of the traumatic event

Resuscitation occurs throughout the primary survey, with problems being treated as soon as they are found: 'treat first what kills first'.

It is essential to adhere to the structured process of AcBCDE. 'Distracting' injuries must not interrupt the primary and secondary surveys or life-threatening injuries may be missed.

Ac – Airway and in-line cervical spine immobilisation

Airway

If c-spine injury is suspected, try to open the airway using the jaw thrust manoeuvre alone while immobilising the cervical spine. Opening the airway takes priority, however, and head

Chapter 11 The Injured Child

extension may be necessary; very gently increase the amount of extension until the airway is open. Take great care! The oropharynx is cleared of debris, blood, vomit and other secretions by gentle suction under direct vision. It may be necessary to assist the airway by using an oropharyngeal airway, remembering that this will not protect the airway in the event of vomiting, as vomit can be inhaled. If the child tolerates an oropharyngeal airway, this indicates loss of the gag reflex and intubation should be considered. In severe trauma, a tracheal tube is used to secure the airway or, when intubation is not possible, a surgical airway is fashioned.

In-line cervical spine immobilisation

Cervical spine injury is uncommon in children. However, if it is missed and the child is incorrectly managed, there can be tragic consequences such as complete paralysis, quadriplegia or death. The cervical spine must be kept in-line in order to minimise the risk of further damage.

Figure 11.1 shows the jaw thrust with the head held in the neutral position and the cervical spine immobilised, without extension or flexion of the head i.e. the cervical spine is kept in-line with the rest of the spine.

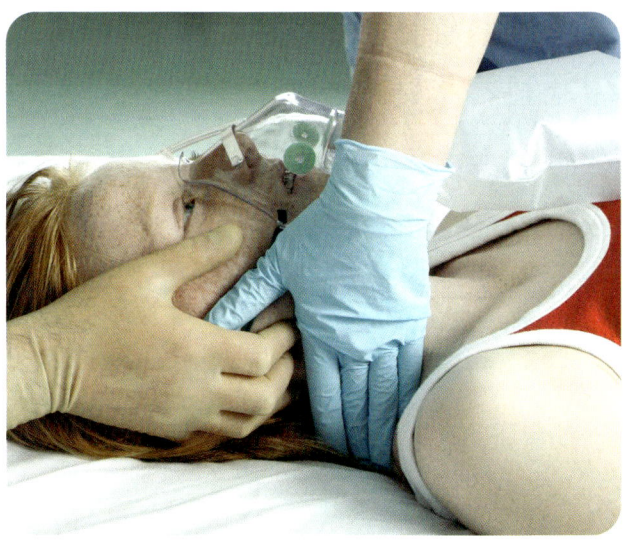

Figure 11.2 Determine correct collar size by measuring the distance from jaw angle to upper trapezius muscle

An assistant should size the correct collar and carefully slide it under the hands of the person maintaining the in-line cervical immobilisation and airway (Figure 11.3).

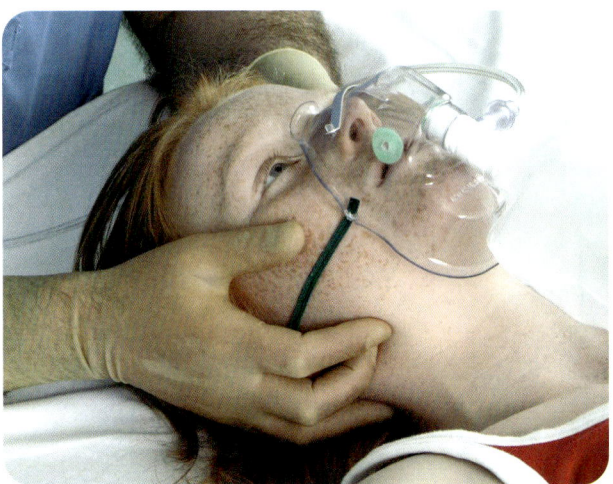

Figure 11.1 Jaw thrust on a child with manual in-line cervical spine immobilisation

Manual in-line cervical immobilisation must be performed until a hard collar and appropriate strapping with head blocks are securely applied.

Sizing the cervical collar

The cervical collar must fit exactly; if it is too small, the head may become flexed on the spine, if too large, the neck may be able to move in any direction and therefore the cervical spine is not immobilised. The manufacturers fitting instructions should be followed but a common method of sizing is described below.

The appropriate collar size is determined by measuring the distance between the angle of the jaw and the upper part of the trapezius while the child's head is in the neutral position (Figure 11.2). The number of fingers that can be comfortably inserted within this space is compared to the markers on the cervical collar.

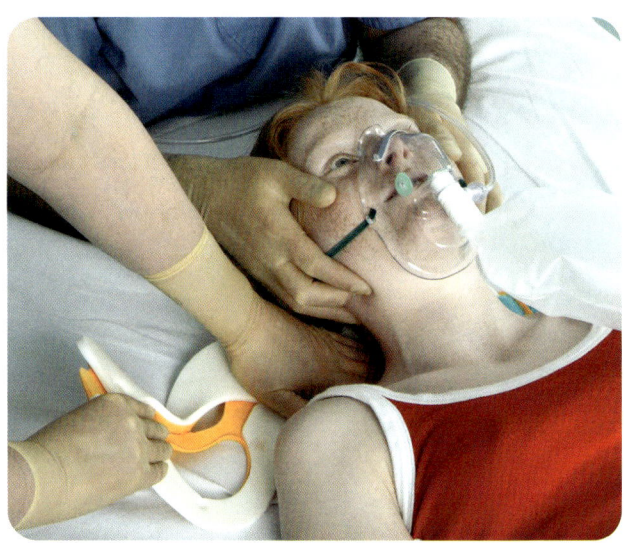

Figure 11.3 The posterior part of the collar is slid under the neck while in-line cervical spine immobilisation is maintained

The collar is fitted around the neck carefully (Figure 11.4) and then fasted. However, before the collar is fastened, the neck is inspected for distended veins, tracheal deviation, wounds or subcutaneous emphysema. If possible use a collar that permits the trachea to be seen and felt.

Hands are placed on the outside of the collar as it is being fastened, maintaining the airway and in-line cervical immobilisation throughout. On either side of the head are placed two head blocks or sand bags. Two straps or strips of adhesive tape are then applied; one across the head of the child and the other over the lower aspect of the cervical collar (Figure 11.5). The ends of the tape are smoothed onto fixed structures that will not move, i.e. not the bed sheet.

EUROPEAN PAEDIATRIC LIFE SUPPORT

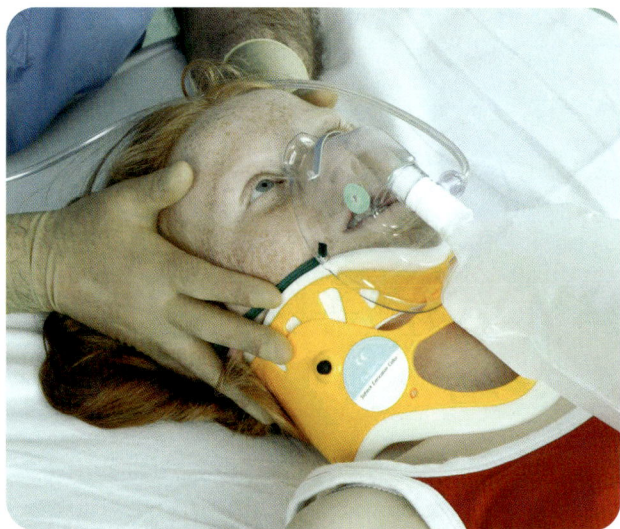

Figure 11.4 The cervical collar is fitted around the neck with cervical spine protection throughout

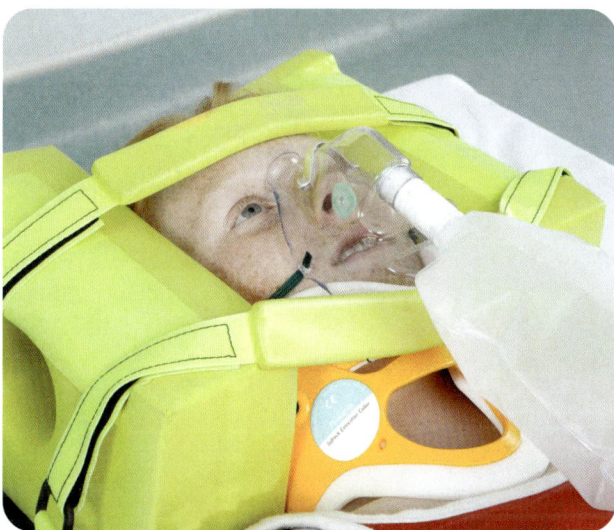

Figure 11.5 The cervical collar is secured. Two straps applied with head blocks placed either side

Only when these manoeuvres have been completed can the immobilising hands be removed.

The in-line cervical spine immobilisation can only be removed when there has been a normal neurological examination. A normal cervical spine x-ray does not guarantee the absence of neurological damage as spinal cord injury without radiological anomaly (SCIWORA) may be present.

B – Breathing and ventilation

The effectiveness of breathing and ventilation must be evaluated after the airway is opened and high-flow oxygen given.

If breathing is ineffective, ventilation must be assisted by BMV with 100% oxygen and tracheal intubation if indicated (Table 11.1). Rarely, a surgical airway may be necessary.

Intubation is a specialist skill and a second person is often required to control the cervical spine during the intubation manoeuvre. This role is vital if the cervical collar and head

> **Table 11.1 Indications for intubation and assisted ventilation**
>
> - Inadequate oxygenation by bag-mask ventilation
> - Respiratory arrest
> - Respiratory failure (hypoventilation and/or hypoxia despite 100% oxygen)
> - Glasgow coma score < 8/15 or 'P' or 'U' on AVPU score
> - Prolonged or controlled ventilation required
> - Flail chest, severe facial injuries, or head injury with seizures
> - Inhalation injury with burns around the mouth or rest of the face, carboneous sputum or a hoarse voice

blocks/sand bags are removed to allow intubation to take place. In-line cervical spine immobilisation without any extension of the neck during intubation is mandatory.

The oral route is preferred for tracheal intubation as the nasotracheal route can lead to neck extension (worsening cervical spine injury), damage to adenoid tissue (with associated haemorrhage) and, in the case of basilar skull fracture, direct damage to the brain.

A rapid sequence intubation with cricoid pressure should be considered as the stomach may be full. If cricoid pressure impedes ventilation or intubation however, it should be removed (Chapter 4).

Hyperventilation

This should not be performed in patients with head injuries as cerebral vasoconstriction induced by hypocapnia aggravates brain ischaemic injuries. The $PaCO_2$ should be maintained in the lower normal range (4.6-6 kPa).

Gastric distension

Significant gastric distension can occur with swallowed air, BMV or from air leak around the tracheal tube. This impairs diaphragmatic movements and affects ventilation. Gastric distension increases the risk of vomiting and aspiration of the stomach contents can occur. A gastric tube should be placed following intubation. The oral route is preferred in cases of craniofacial trauma (owing to the risk of maxillofacial or basilar skull fractures). The position of the orogastric or nasogastric tube must be checked after insertion.

C – Circulation and haemorrhage control

The assessment of cardiovascular status and restoration of normal circulating volume are the key elements of managing a child with haemorrhagic/hypovolaemic shock; hence two routes of vascular access must be secured in children who have suffered severe trauma. At the same time, blood samples for cross-match and laboratory studies must be taken. Wear gloves in all circumstances. Protective clothing and goggles may also be worn.

Blood loss is the commonest cause of shock in injured children. Blood loss can be visible (i.e. external) or hidden (i.e. internal). Children with burns lose fluids from the burned surface.

Traumatic haemorrhage

Any obvious exsanguinating blood loss from a blood vessel must be controlled by direct pressure, using a thin layer of gauze, even when the amount lost seems small. This is because there may initially be protective vasoconstriction. Haemostatic forceps and tourniquets should not be used except in cases of uncontrolled haemorrhage from traumatic amputation.

Open fractures can cause large quantities of blood to be lost. Splinting of limb fractures (re-establishing normal anatomical position) reduces blood loss, pain and tissue damage.

Pelvic fractures or major long bone closed fractures may also be associated with soft tissue damage and the extravasation of blood. If hypovolaemia persists despite control of external haemorrhage, and the need for fluid resuscitation persists, internal haemorrhage must be excluded. Many centres use rapid ultrasound examination e.g. focused assessment with sonography for trauma (FAST) for this purpose. Surgical involvement in the management of any trauma case is mandatory.

Causes of internal haemorrhage

Intrathoracic, retroperitoneal (associated with pelvic fractures) and intra-abdominal bleeding are causes of life-threatening internal haemorrhage.

Intra-abdominal haemorrhage (associated with a laceration of an organ such as the spleen or liver) can present with peritonism, abdominal distension (which does not decompress with a gastric tube) and signs of circulatory failure and/or shock. Blood or bile-stained aspirates via the nasal or orogastric route are also suggestive of abdominal bleeding and damage.

Intra-abdominal bleeding, however, may show few signs, hence there must be a high index of suspicion, especially if there is a history of abdominal trauma.

Isolated closed fracture of a long bone can be associated with blood loss but it is rarely associated with hypovolaemic shock. Closed head trauma is not associated with hypovolaemia and another source of bleeding must be sought if hypovolaemic shock is present in a child with head injuries.

Evaluation of blood loss

Evaluation of blood loss (and category of hypovolaemic shock) depends on assessment of respiratory rate, volume of the peripheral pulses, peripheral perfusion (capillary refill time and skin temperature), level of consciousness and BP.

Volume of blood loss relates to the changes in these signs. Hypovolaemic shock can be graded on a scale of I to IV, with Grade I being the mildest and IV the severest (Table 11.2). Decompensated circulatory failure is apparent from Grade III hypovolaemic shock.

The child should be reassessed repeatedly as there may be rapid alterations in the circulatory status, such as the development of internal haemorrhage (e.g. intra-abdominal bleeding). Response to treatment must also be assessed to see if further interventions are required.

Vascular access

The mainstay of treatment for hypovolaemic shock is intravascular fluid replacement. Circulatory access can be achieved by the placement of two peripheral short wide-bore cannulae, or as IO access as usually IV and IO routes are the fastest ways to gain access (Chapter 5).

Treatment of hypovolaemic shock

In mild to moderate hypovolaemic shock (Grades I-II) a bolus of 20 ml kg^{-1} of crystalloid or colloid is given. The child must be reassessed and if signs of shock remain, a second bolus of 20 ml kg^{-1} of fluids is administered. If the child remains shocked, 10 ml kg^{-1} of warmed blood should be given; the administration of cold blood causes hypothermia and hyperkalemia. Grade III and IV hypovolaemic shock require the immediate infusion of 40 ml kg^{-1} of crystalloid or colloid followed by blood (as above). If type-specific or full cross-match blood is not available within 10 minutes, then Group O Rhesus-negative blood should be used.

Table 11.2 Clinical signs of grades of hypovolaemic shock (as percentage of circulating blood volume)

	Grade I-II	Grade III	Grade IV
Blood loss	< 25 %	25-40 %	> 40 %
Heart rate	Mildly increased	Moderately increased	Tachycardia/bradycardia
Systolic blood pressure	Normal or increased	Normal or decreased	Decreased
Peripheral pulse volume	Normal/Reduced	Moderately reduced	Severely reduced
Capillary refill time	Normal/increased	Moderately increased	Severely increased
Peripheral skin temperature	Cool, pale	Cold, mottled	Cold, pale
Respiratory rate	Moderately increased	Severely increased	Sighing respiration Agonal breathing
Mental status	Mild Agitation	Lethargic	Reacts only to pain unconscious

Although intraabdominal bleeding can often be managed conservatively, surgery may be indicated when repeated transfusions are needed to maintain normal physiological parameters. An experienced surgeon must decide whether operative intervention is needed to stop internal bleeding.

Hypertonic saline and delayed fluid resuscitation for hypotensive injured children are not recommended.

D – Disability

The child's disability is determined from his level of consciousness according to the AVPU scale, posture and examination of the pupils for size, symmetry and response to light.

AVPU relates the response (level of consciousness) of the child to a stimulus as follows:

- **A** for ALERT
- **V** for VOICE
- **P** for PAIN
- **U** for UNRESPONSIVE to painful stimulus

An AVPU score of P (i.e. response to pain) is equivalent to a score of 8 on the Glasgow coma score when protective gag reflexes are lost. There is, therefore, a risk of aspiration of the stomach contents at this level of consciousness and tracheal intubation must be considered to protect the airway.

The pupils must be examined for size and direct response to light. A unilateral dilated pupil in association with head injury may indicate an intracranial bleed on the same side and requires urgent neurological referral. The child's posture must be noted: the arms flexed towards the trunk represents decorticate abnormality, whereas if the child's arms are extended, this may indicate decerebrate pathology. Both of these postures are worrying and the underlying cause must be treated.

The child's vital signs and neurological status must be recorded on a regular basis and the results interpreted in the context of the child's clinical state.

The goal in the primary survey is to diagnose severe head injury which may require urgent neurosurgical intervention, and/or may determine the need for specific intensive care techniques.

E – Exposure

The child's clothes should be removed in an appropriate manner so that any injuries can be seen in the secondary survey.

As the child has a large body surface to weight ratio, heat loss occurs relatively quickly and he should be covered when the secondary survey has been completed. Warming devices e.g. overhead radiant heaters and warming blankets, should be used to keep the child warm. Marked hypothermia can be deleterious.

Secondary survey

The secondary survey is a full examination to detect occult injury. The child's entire body (head-to-toe) is examined back and front by undertaking a log-roll.

Further details about the mechanism of injury which relates to the impacting force is important in managing the child should be sought.

The secondary survey should only start when all immediate life-threatening injuries have been treated. The vital signs relating to AcBCDE should be regularly assessed during and after the secondary survey; deterioration in the child's clinical signs requires the primary and then the secondary survey to be repeated, stopping to deal with any abnormal clinical features as they are found. In the pre-hospital setting, examination should be limited to the primary survey to exclude life-threatening injuries before and during transportation to the hospital.

Log-roll

The purpose of the log-roll is to keep the child's spine in-line with the rest of his body while his back is examined.

The number of people required to perform a log-roll is four for a child and three for an infant depending on the child's size (Figure 11.6). Each member of the log-roll team must know his role. This should be confirmed by the team leader who is the person performing the in-line cervical spine immobilisation. Clear instructions about moving the child are given by the team leader. An additional person is required to examine the back of the child, from the head to the thorax and abdomen, feeling along the spine, inspecting the anus (which includes a rectal examination to exclude spinal cord injury), performing a vaginal examination (if appropriate) and finishing with the back of the legs.

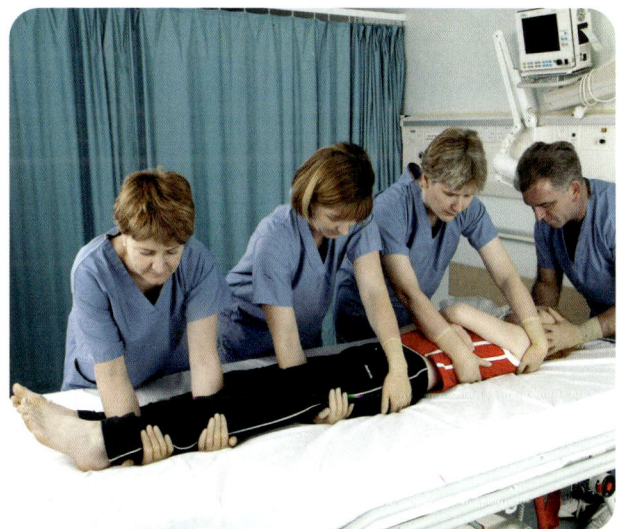

Figure 11.6 Log-roll hand positions

When the survey is complete, the examiner makes it clear that the examination has finished. The controlled return of the child to the supine position is led by the team leader.

The child should be told what is happening even if he appears to be unconscious. The need for full exposure should be made clear but the child's dignity must be maintained.

X-rays

Routine radiological investigations are carried out at the end of the primary survey, namely:

- Chest
- Pelvis
- Cervical spine x-ray may be deferred as part of the secondary survey

X-ray of any limb injury must wait until the child is stable and the secondary survey has been completed. These x-rays of the limbs should have an anterior-posterior view as well as lateral view so as not to miss any fractures.

History

A short history informs the management of the child and can be remembered by the acronym **AMPLE** (Table 11.3).

Table 11.3 AMPLE for history taking in secondary survey

A	Allergy
M	Medication
P	Past medical history
L	Last meal
E	Environment (history of accident, mechanism of injury

Allergy, especially to drugs that may be used e.g. penicillin, must be asked about and details of current **medications**, e.g. if the child has a chronic illness such as epilepsy, diabetes or asthma. The drugs used in these conditions may have an impact on the child's management. The child's **past medical history** may explain some of the physical signs such as cerebral palsy, although injury must be excluded. The closer the injury to the time of the **last meal** the greater the risk of vomiting and potential aspiration; cricoid pressure may be required to protect the airway during intubation (Chapter 4). Asking about **environment/events** gives information about the energy involved in the injury and potential clinical consequences.

Emergency treatment

Emergency treatments for abnormalities found in the secondary survey must be identified and managed as soon as possible after life-threatening injuries are treated.

Analgesia and sedation

This is an essential part of the management of the injured child. Beware of hypoxia, hypovolaemia or hypoglycaemia which can cause symptoms such as aggression or altered level of consciousness.

Definitive Care

Definitive care is the final part of the structured approach to trauma. Good note-taking and appropriate referral are essential in providing optimum treatment. If definitive care is to be undertaken in a specialist centre, transfer will be necessary.

Transfer

The transferring team should contact the receiving hospital about the clinical state of the child giving details of suspected injuries, AMPLE, and any procedures or treatments which have been carried out.

The expected time of arrival and the need for additional specialists must be communicated early to ensure their availability. The transferring team must be able to deal with any problem arising during transportation e.g. deteriorating airway, inadequate ventilation or circulatory problems. External haemorrhage must be controlled before and during transfer and there must be secure intravenous or intraosseous access. The AcBCDE parameters must be evaluated and monitored throughout. When indicated, the transfer should be instigated without delay. Unnecessary examinations and treatments should be avoided, providing the child can be safely transported without deteriorating en route.

The optimal trauma team consists of a paediatric anaesthetist, paediatric intensivist, emergency physician (ideally a paediatric emergency specialist), experienced paediatric surgeon and paediatric trauma nurses. The most experienced clinician in paediatric trauma should act as team leader. Other specialists may be involved particularly after the secondary survey, e.g. a neurosurgical opinion if there is evidence of injury to the brain.

Brain injuries

Brain injuries are responsible for 70% of deaths in the first 48 hours following paediatric trauma.

Assessment

- History of injury (mechanism of injury, loss of consciousness, headache, vomiting, amnesia, seizures)
- General assessment (AcBCDE), bruises, lacerations, fractures, bleeding from ears and nose or focal neurological pathology
- AcBCDE reassessment should be carried out on a regular basis

Treatment

Primary brain damage occurs at the time of the trauma and is generally irreversible.

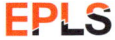

Aggressive treatment must be given to prevent secondary brain damage which may be due to:

- Hypoxia from hypoventilation, airway obstruction, pulmonary contusion, aspiration or seizures (with or without hypoglycaemia)

- Ischaemia which is associated with hypotension, focal/generalised cerebral oedema, extradural/subdural haematoma

Hypoxia should be prevented by adequate BMV with 100% oxygen and, if indicated, early recourse to tracheal intubation. The underlying cause of hypoxia must also be treated.

Secondary brain damage can also be prevented by avoiding systemic hypotension and by treating raised intracranial pressure. Both hypoglycaemia and hyperglycaemia can also worsen the outcome, hence careful bedside blood glucose monitoring is essential.

Raised intracranial pressure

Raised intracranial pressure (RICP), e.g. from cerebral oedema, can lead to herniation of the brain through the foramen magnum causing death as the skull has limited ability to expand. It should be identified (ideally prevented) and treated rapidly. It is clinically indicated by elevated systemic BP, bradycardia and 'sighing' respirations (this is called Cushing's triad).

Steps to diminish the likelihood of RICP:

1. The internal jugular veins should not be cannulated for central venous access, as this hinders venous drainage from the brain.

2. The head and chest can be slightly elevated (15-45°), provided there is no evidence of systemic hypotension, to aid venous drainage. Flexion of the body when achieving elevation should be avoided to protect the spinal cord. In case of hypotension, the patient must be kept flat to optimise systemic arterial BP.

3. Mean arterial pressure must be maintained at or above the normal value for the age to preserve cerebral perfusion pressure.

4. The $PaCO_2$ should be kept between 4.6-6.0 kPa (i.e. within the normal range). Hyperventilation should only be carried out under careful supervision if there is RICP.

5. Mannitol must be given if there is evidence of RICP. This can be given at 0.25 g kg^{-1} IV or IO over 20 min with repeated doses up to 1 g kg^{-1}. Urinary output monitoring is essential and urinary catheterisation is required (via the suprapubic route if there is urethral trauma). Hypertonic saline is used as an alternative therapy.

6. Hyperglycaemia and hypoglycaemia must be avoided.

7. Seizures should be treated with benzodiazepines and antiepileptic medication as required.

Hypovolaemic shock in brain injuries

Isolated closed head injuries do not usually cause hypovolaemic shock and internal haemorrhage must be considered as a cause. Other causes such as intrathoracic or intra-abdominal trauma, pelvic and long bone fractures must be ruled out. Scalp lacerations, and in certain cases acute extradural haemorrhage in the newborn, can lead to a significant blood loss so the scalp must be carefully inspected.

The most common cause of death in trauma is hypovolaemic shock; hypovolaemic shock due to rapid blood loss is a faster cause of death than RICP. Fluid and blood transfusions to treat hypovolaemia are essential, even though there may already be brain injury.

Investigations of cerebral lesions

Haemodynamically stable patients can have CT scans of the brain. However, resuscitation equipment and a resuscitation team must be on hand as the seemingly stabilised patient can suddenly deteriorate.

A CT scan may demonstrate treatable conditions such as:

- Skull fractures (compound and depressed, including basilar skull fractures associated with 0.4-5% risk infection)

- Intracranial haemorrhages (extradural haematoma, subdural haematoma, cerebral contusions and subarachnoid haemorrhage)

- Midline shift of white and grey matter

- Signs of cerebral oedema and RICP (absent sulci, slit-like cerebral ventricles)

Extradural haematoma

Extradural haematomas are life-threatening emergencies requiring extremely urgent drainage. A rapidly expanding extradural haematoma can cause cerebral herniation.

Systemic arterial hypertension

Systemic hypertension associated with bradycardia and irregular respiration (Cushing's triad) suggests RICP. The systemic hypertension should not be treated with antihypertensive agents but RICP should be managed appropriately.

Hyperglycaemia

Hyperglycaemia aggravates ischaemic cerebral lesions. Administration of glucose-containing solutions must be avoided during resuscitation, unless to treat documented hypoglycaemia. Monitoring of blood sugar levels is mandatory.

Chest trauma (primary survey)

Life-threatening conditions such as tension pneumothorax, massive haemothorax, flail chest and cardiac tamponade can be identified and treated during the primary survey. If the child deteriorates during the secondary survey, or later due to one of these conditions, the primary survey must be repeated.

Pneumothorax

Pneumothorax means that there is air, between the lung and the internal thoracic wall, which compresses the lung and impedes ventilation.

There are three mains types – simple, tension and open. Respiratory failure can be caused by all three.

All forms of pneumothorax can be diagnosed clinically.

Simple pneumothorax

This represents a limited air leak into the pleural space which causes the lung to collapse without there being significant haemodynamic signs.

A small simple pneumothorax may only be identified on secondary survey and chest x-ray. It may be managed conservatively provided there is continuous monitoring of the child's physiological parameters to ensure there is no deterioration in the clinical condition. Immediate chest drainage is however mandatory, if the child requires ventilation. This is because the simple pneumothorax could be converted into a tension pneumothorax.

Tension pneumothorax

When air is forced into the pleural cavity (a limited space) without means of escape, it accumulates and comes under pressure. This pressure can displace the mediastinum to the opposite side of the chest causing compression of the great vessels, so interfering with venous return, causing obstructive shock with a concomitant fall in systemic BP. The jugular venous pressure is raised if there is no associated hypovolaemia.

Signs:

- Hypoxia
- Absent/decreased breath sounds on affected side
- Neck vein distension
- Tracheal deviation away from the side of the tension pneumothorax

Treatment:

1. Airway opening.
2. Oxygen (100%) by face mask or BMV.
3. Needle thoracocentesis – the insertion of a cannula into the second intercostal space in the midclavicular line on the side of the tension pneumothorax. When the needle of the cannula is removed, a hiss of escaping air is heard as the pressure within the pleural space is released. The cannula is left to vent the air.
4. Chest drain insertion should be undertaken as soon as possible, provided it doesn't delay progressing the assessment and management of the patient.

If the child deteriorates at any stage following the needle thoracocentesis, air may have reaccumulated, reforming the tension pneumothorax. This may be due to the cannula kinking. Needle thoracocentesis must be repeated and a chest drain inserted as soon as possible.

Open pneumothorax

Open pneumothorax results from a penetrating chest wound and makes a sucking noise. When the child breathes in, a negative intrathoracic pressure is generated (which normally draws air into the lungs with each inspiration) and air rushes in through the wound into the pleural space.

Signs:

- Penetrating chest wound (examine front and back)
- Audible air passage through the wound
- Decreased chest wall movement on affected side
- Decreased breath sounds on affected side
- Increased percussion noted on affected side
- A tension pneumothorax can develop from an open pneumothorax

Treatment:

1. Airway opening.
2. Oxygen (100%) by face mask or BMV.
3. Close the defect with an occlusive dressing taped on three sides, to allow entrapped air to escape while exhaling and impeding air entry when breathing in.
4. Chest drain insertion on the same side as the pneumothorax but in an area away from the wound.

If a tension pneumothorax is present, treat accordingly. If positive pressure ventilation is required, chest drain placement is mandatory and should be sited as soon as possible.

Massive haemothorax

This is due to blood accumulating in the thoracic cavity as a result of a pulmonary parenchymal injury associated with pulmonary vessels or chest wall injuries.

A haemothorax may contain a significant proportion of a child's total circulatory blood volume.

Signs:

- Hypoxia
- Hypovolaemic shock
- Decreased chest wall movements on affected side
- Decreased breath sounds on affected side
- Decreased percussion noted on affected side
- Neck veins may be flat, not full or distended

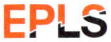

usually happens in term infants in utero before delivery. A large randomised trial has shown no advantage to suctioning the airway whilst the head is on the perineum and this may delay resuscitation. This practice is, therefore, no longer recommended. If the baby is vigorous after birth through meconium, a randomised trial has shown that suctioning at any time offers no advantage and no specific action (other than drying and wrapping the baby) is needed. If the baby has absent or inadequate respirations, a heart rate < 100 min^{-1} or hypotonia, inspect the oropharynx with a laryngoscope and aspirate any particulate meconium seen using a wide-bore catheter. If intubation is possible and the baby is still unresponsive, aspirate the trachea using either a wide-bore suction catheter or the tracheal tube. However, if intubation cannot be achieved immediately, clear the oropharynx and start mask inflation. If, while attempting to clear the airway, the heart rate falls to < 60 min^{-1} then stop airway clearance, give inflation breaths and start ventilating the baby.

Breathing (aeration breaths and ventilation)

The first 5 breaths in term babies should be inflation breaths in order to replace lung fluid in the alveoli with air. These should be 2-3-second sustained breaths using a continuous gas supply, a pressure-limiting device and a mask. Use a transparent, circular soft mask big enough to cover the nose and mouth of the baby. If no such system is available, or you are not familiar with it, then a 500-ml self-inflating bag and a blow-off valve set at 30-40 cmH$_2$O can be used. This is especially useful if compressed air or oxygen is not available.

The chest may not move during the first 1-3 breaths as fluid is displaced. Adequate ventilation is usually indicated by either a rapidly increasing heart rate or a heart rate that is maintained at > 100 min^{-1}. Therefore, reassess the heart rate after delivery of the first 5 breaths. It is safe to assume the chest has been successfully inflated if the heart rate responds. Once the chest is inflated and the heart rate has increased or the chest has been seen to move, ventilation should be continued at a rate of 30-40 min^{-1}. Continue ventilatory support until regular breathing is established. Where possible, start resuscitation of the baby at birth with air. There is now good evidence for this in term babies and oxygen toxicity is a real concern with premature babies. Use of supplemental oxygen should be guided by pulse oximetry with reasonable levels listed (Table 12.2) and on the algorithm.

If the heart rate has not responded then check for chest movement rather than auscultation as in fluid-filled lungs, breath sounds may be heard without lung inflation. Go back and check airway opening manoeuvres and repeat the inflation breaths.

Circulation

If the heart rate remains slow or absent, despite adequate ventilation for 30 seconds as shown by chest movement, then chest compressions should be started. Chest compressions will help to move oxygenated blood from the lungs to the heart and coronary arteries. The blood you move can only be oxygenated if the lungs have air in them. In the newly born baby, cardiac compromise is always the result of respiratory failure and can only be effectively treated if effective ventilation is occurring.

The most efficient way of delivering chest compressions in the neonate is to encircle the chest with both hands, so that the fingers lie behind the baby and the thumbs are apposed on the sternum just below the inter-nipple line (Figure 12.6). Compress the chest briskly, by one third of its depth. In newborn babies, current advice is to perform three compressions for each ventilation breath (3:1 ratio).

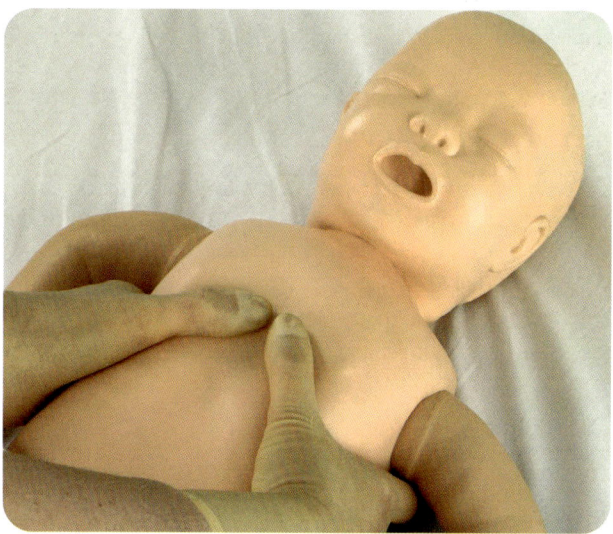

Figure 12.6 Chest compression on an infant: Two-thumb encircling technique

The purpose of chest compression is to move oxygenated blood or drugs to the coronary arteries in order to initiate cardiac recovery. Thus there is no point in starting chest compression before effective lung inflation has been established. Similarly, compressions are ineffective unless interposed by ventilation breaths of good quality. Therefore, the emphasis must be upon good-quality breaths, followed by effective compressions. Simultaneous delivery of compressions and breaths should be avoided, as the former will reduce the effectiveness of the breaths. It is usually only necessary to continue chest compressions for about 20-30 seconds before the heart responds with an increase in heart rate, so reassess after this period.

Once the heart rate is > 60 min^{-1} and rising, chest compression can be discontinued. Maintain ventilations until effective breathing or mechanical ventilation is established.

Drugs

If after adequate lung inflation and cardiac compression the heart rate has not responded, drug therapy should be considered. However, the most common reason for failure of the heart rate to respond is failure to achieve lung inflation, and there is no point in giving drugs unless the airway is open and the lungs have been inflated. Airway and breathing must be reassessed as adequate before proceeding to drug therapy. Venous access will be required via an umbilical venous line (or rarely through an intraosseus needle). The outcome is poor if drugs are required for resuscitation.

Adrenaline

The alpha-adrenergic effect of adrenaline (epinephrine) increases coronary artery perfusion during resuscitation, enhancing oxygen delivery to the heart. In the presence of profound unresponsive bradycardia or circulatory standstill, 10 mcg kg^{-1} (0·1 ml kg^{-1} 1:10000) adrenaline (epinephrine) may be given intravenously. Further doses of 10-30 mcg kg^{-1} (0·1-0·3 ml 1:10000) may be tried at 3-5-minute intervals if there is no response. The tracheal route cannot be recommended as there are insufficient data. However, if it is given via the tracheal route it is likely that doses of at least 50 mcg kg^{-1} will be required to achieve a similar effect to intravenous. Such an unproven administration should not compromise airway and breathing management or obtaining umbilical access.

Bicarbonate

Any baby who is in terminal apnoea will have a significant metabolic acidosis. Acidosis depresses cardiac function. Bicarbonate 1-2 mmol kg^{-1} (2-4 ml kg^{-1} of 4·2% solution) may be used to raise the pH and enhance the effects of oxygen and epinephrine.

Bicarbonate use remains controversial and it should only be used in the absence of discernible cardiac output despite all resuscitative efforts or in profound and unresponsive bradycardia.

Glucose

Hypoglycaemia is a potential problem for all stressed or asphyxiated babies. It is treated using a slow bolus of 2.5 ml kg^{-1} of 10% glucose intravenously, and then providing a secure intravenous glucose infusion at a rate of 100 ml kg^{-1} day^{-1} of 10% glucose. BM stix are not reliable in neonates when reading < 5 mmol l^{-1}.

Fluid

Very occasionally hypovolaemia may be present because of known or suspected blood loss (antepartum haemorrhage, placenta or vasa praevia, unclamped cord) or it may be secondary to loss of vascular tone following asphyxia. Volume expansion, initially with 10 ml kg^{-1}, may be appropriate. Saline (0.9%) can be used; alternatively colloidal gelatine has been used safely and if blood loss is acute and severe, non-cross-matched O-negative blood should be given immediately. However, most newborn or neonatal resuscitations do not require fluid unless there has been known blood loss or septicaemic shock.

Naloxone

This is not a drug of resuscitation. Occasionally, a baby who has been effectively resuscitated – is pink, with a heart rate > 100 min^{-1} – may not breathe spontaneously because of the effects of maternal opiates. If respiratory depressant effects are suspected the baby should be given naloxone intramuscularly (200 mcg in a full term baby). Smaller doses of 10 mcg kg^{-1} will also reverse the sedation but the effect will only last a short time (20 minutes IV or a few hours IM). Intravenous naloxone has a half-life shorter than opiates, and there is no evidence to recommend intra-tracheal administration.

Response to resuscitation

The first indication of success will be an increase in heart rate. Recovery of respiratory drive may be delayed. Babies in terminal apnoea will tend to gasp first as they recover before starting normal respirations. Those who were in primary apnoea are likely to start with normal breaths, which may commence at any stage of resuscitation.

Tracheal intubation

Most babies can be resuscitated using a mask system. Swedish data suggests that if this is applied adequately, only 1:500 babies may actually need intubation. However, tracheal intubation, if it is performed, is especially useful in prolonged resuscitations, pre-term babies and meconium aspiration. It should be considered if mask ventilation has failed, although the most common reason for failure with mask ventilation is poor positioning of the head with consequent failure to open the airway or poor application of the mask resulting in a leak.

The technique of intubation is the same as for infants and is described in Chapter 4. A normal full-term newborn usually needs a 3·5-mm tracheal tube, but 4·0-, 3·0- and 2·5-mm tubes should also be available.

Tracheal tube placement must be assessed visually during intubation and in most cases will be confirmed by a rapid response in heart rate on ventilating via the tracheal tube. If in doubt exhaled CO_2 detection will correctly identify most correctly sited tubes in the presence of any cardiac output. Detection of exhaled carbon dioxide should be used to confirm tracheal tube placement along with chest x-ray.

Special Cases

Pre-term babies

Unexpected deliveries outside delivery suites are more likely to be premature. Premature babies are more likely to get cold (higher surface area to mass ratio), and more likely to become hypoglycaemic (fewer glycogen stores). There are now several trials which support the use of plastic bags placed over babies of < 29 weeks' gestation or < 1000 g before drying in order to keep them warm. The babies should then be placed under a radiant heater. The effectiveness of this technique without a radiant heater has not been tested in a trial.

The more premature a baby the less likely it is to establish adequate respirations. Preterm babies < 32 weeks gestation are likely to be deficient in surfactant especially after unexpected or precipitate delivery. The surfactant, secreted by pneumocytes in the alveolar epithelium, reduces alveolar surface tension and prevents alveolar collapse on expiration. Small amounts of surfactant can be demonstrated from

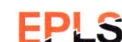

about 20 weeks' gestation, but a surge in production occurs at 30-34 weeks. Surfactant is released at birth due to aeration and distension of the alveoli. The half-life of the surfactant is approximately 12 hours. Production is reduced by hypothermia (< 35 °C), hypoxia and acidosis (pH < 7·25). In babies born before 32 weeks, one must anticipate a lack of surfactant. The effort of respiration will be increased, although the musculature will be less developed. They may require help to establish prompt aeration and ventilation, and may subsequently require exogenous surfactant therapy.

The lungs of pre-term babies are more fragile than those of term babies and thus are much more susceptible to damage from over-distension. Therefore, it is appropriate to start with a lower inflation pressure of 2·0-2·5 kPa (20-25 cmH$_2$O) but do not be afraid to increase this to 30 cmH$_2$O if there is no heart rate response.

It should be noted that very obvious chest wall movement in premature babies of < 28 weeks gestation may indicate excessive and potentially damaging tidal volumes.

Premature babies are more susceptible to the toxic effects of hyperoxia. Using a pulse oximeter to monitor both heart rate and oxygen saturation in these babies from birth makes stabilisation much easier. Exposing babies at birth to high concentrations of oxygen can have significant adverse longer term effects. Ranges of pre-ductal oxygen saturation found in the first few minutes of life in well preterm infants are increasingly being reported however, normal values in well babies born before 32 weeks gestation are based upon small numbers. Therefore, at present, additional oxygen should not be given if the oxygen saturation from the right arm or wrist is above the values, in Table 12.2.

Actions in the event of poor initial response to resuscitation

1. Check airway and breathing.

2. Check for a technical fault.

   (a) Is mask ventilation effective? Observe movement.

   (b) Is the tracheal tube in the trachea? Auscultate both axillae, listen at the mouth for a large leak, and observe movement. Use an exhaled CO$_2$ detector to ensure tracheal tube position.

   (c) Is the tracheal tube in the right bronchus? Auscultate both axillae and observe movement.

   (d) Is the tracheal tube blocked? If there is doubt about the position or patency of the tracheal tube re-place it. Use an exhaled CO$_2$ detector.

   (e) Is a longer inflation time required?

   (f) If starting in air then increase the oxygen concentration. This is least likely to be a cause, although if monitoring saturations it could be a cause for slow increase.

3. Does the baby have a pneumothorax? This occurs spontaneously in up to 1% of newborns, but those needing action in the delivery unit are exceptionally rare. Auscultate the chest for asymmetry of breath sounds. A cold light source can be used to transilluminate the chest – a pneumothorax may show as a hyper-illuminating area. If a tension pneumothorax is thought to be present clinically, a 21-gauge butterfly needle should be inserted through the second intercostal space in the mid-clavicular line. Alternatively, a 22-gauge cannula connected to a three-way tap may be used. Remember that you may well cause a pneumothorax during this procedure.

4. Does the baby remain cyanosed despite breathing with a good heart rate? There may be a congenital heart malformation, which may be duct-dependent or a persistent pulmonary hypertension.

5. If, after resuscitation, the baby is pink and has a good heart rate but is not breathing effectively, it may be suffering the effects of maternal opiates. Naloxone 200 mcg IM may be considered. This should outlast the opiate effect.

6. Is there severe anaemia or hypovolaemia? In case of large blood loss, 20 ml kg^{-1} O-negative blood or a volume expander should be given.

Birth outside the delivery room

Whenever a baby is born unexpectedly, a great difficulty often lies in keeping it warm. Drying and wrapping, turning up the heating and closing windows and doors are all important in maintaining the body temperature. Special care must be taken to clamp and cut the cord to prevent blood loss.

Hospitals with emergency departments should have guidelines for resuscitation at birth, summoning help and post-resuscitation transfer of babies born within the department.

Babies born unexpectedly, outside hospital, will be at greater risk of being pre-term and of getting cold. However, the principles of resuscitation are identical to the hospital setting. Transport will need to be discussed according to local guidelines.

Post-resuscitation care

Newborns requiring resuscitation may remain unstable or deteriorate. Once adequate ventilation and circulation have been established, the infant should be admitted to a specialised unit, where further monitoring and treatment can be provided.

Hypoglycaemia is associated with adverse neurological outcome, so blood glucose should be maintained in the normal range.

In babies with significant asphyxia during delivery there is now sufficient evidence of improved outcome to recommend

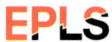

therapeutic hypothermia. It is important to maintain a register of babies receiving this treatment modality. Therapeutic cooling should only be undertaken in centres with experience and the availability of EEG interpretation. Always discuss such babies with the regional network centre at the earliest opportunity.

Passive cooling: Once a decision has been made to offer cooling, if equipment for active cooling is not available, passive cooling can be started while arrangements are made to transfer the baby to a cooling centre.

Avoid hyperthermia: Hyperthermia, particularly induced by external heating, is to be avoided at all costs in babies who have suffered perinatal brain injury.

Discontinuation of resuscitation

The outcome for a baby with no detectable cardiac output for more than 10 minutes is likely to be very poor. Stopping resuscitation early, or not starting resuscitation at all, may be appropriate in situations of extreme prematurity (< 23 weeks), birth weight of < 400 g, or in the presence of lethal abnormalities such as anencephaly or confirmed trisomy 13 or 18.

Resuscitation is nearly always indicated in conditions with a high survival rate and acceptable morbidity. Such decisions should be taken by a senior member of the team, ideally a consultant in consultation with the parents and other team members. In such situations it is therefore essential to summon appropriate help as early as possible.

Communication with the parents

It is important that the team caring for the newborn baby informs the parents of the progress whenever possible. This is likely to be most difficult in unexpected deliveries so prior planning to cover the eventuality may be helpful. Decisions at the end of life must involve the parents whenever possible. All communication should be documented after the event.

Equipment

Face masks

Face masks used for ventilation of the newborn should have a broad soft rim to form a seal against the baby's face. The mask should fit comfortably over the baby's nose and mouth without pressing into his eye sockets or overlapping the chin (Chapter 4).

Effective positive pressure ventilation through a mask can be achieved with either a flow-inflating or self-inflating bag, or with a T-piece mechanical device designed to regulate pressure.

Self-inflating bags

Self-inflating bags used for newborn resuscitation should all have a pressure limiting valve. These blow-off valves can be deliberately overridden during use, but this is rarely necessary. In some cases these valves can be locked in a non-functioning position so it is vital to test them before use. It is important to remember that the blow-off valves of self-inflating bags are flow dependent, and pressures generated by squeezing may exceed those specified by the manufacturer quite easily. Some bags have optional attachments that allow the device to maintain a positive end expiratory pressure (PEEP).

T-pieces

Variable inflation pressures and longer inspiratory times are achieved more consistently in mechanical models when using T-piece devices. These devices also allow more consistent use of PEEP.

Flow-inflating bags

Flow-inflating ('anaesthetic') bags, if used with a pressure monitoring device, can provide both variable inflation pressures and PEEP. They can also provide longer inspiratory times. More training is needed to deliver appropriate pressures using flow-inflating bags compared with T-piece devices or self-inflating bags. There is no evidence that operators can assess lung resistance.

Laryngeal mask airway

The laryngeal mask airway (LMA) has been used successfully in the resuscitation of term and near-term newborns. There are little data on its use and effectiveness when chest compressions are needed, in small preterm newborns or those with meconium stained amniotic fluid. It has been suggested that the LMA, when used by appropriately trained healthcare professionals, may be an effective alternative in establishing an airway in the resuscitation of the newborn, especially if BMV is ineffective or tracheal intubation fails. However, routine use of the LMA in an emergency delivery cannot be currently recommended.

Oxygen administration

If possible start resuscitation with air in all babies. In term babies receiving resuscitation at birth with positive pressure ventilation, it is best to begin with air rather than 100% oxygen. If, despite effective ventilation, there is no increase in heart rate or if oxygenation (guided by pulse oximetry) remains unacceptable (see acceptable values), use of a higher concentration of oxygen should be considered. However, if only 100% oxygen is available then this should be used and resuscitation should not be delayed.

Transportation of the newborn

Following resuscitation of the newborn, continuous monitoring and anticipation of possible complications must continue throughout transportation to a neonatal unit.

Newborns transferred under controlled conditions by skilled healthcare professionals arrive at their destination in better clinical condition. They are significantly warmer, less hypotensive and less acidotic on arrival than if transferred by an inexperienced team; mortality, morbidity and duration of intensive care stay are also reduced. Throughout the transport phase, vital signs must be continuously monitored.

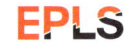

During transport, particular attention should be paid to the risk of accidental extubation or the displacement of chest drains, if present. Tracheal tubes and vascular access must be carefully secured. Hypothermia and hypoglycaemia must be avoided. Family members should be provided with adequate communication and support.

> ### Key learning points
>
> - Most babies need no more than drying, keeping warm and given to mother.
> - The key to successful resuscitation at birth is lung inflation.
> - Start resuscitation with air – only add oxygen if SpO_2 remains low despite good lung inflation.

Further reading

Newborn Life Support Manual 2011, Resuscitation Council UK

Part 11: Neonatal Resuscitation: 2010 International Consensus on Cardiopulmonary Resuscitation and Emergency Cardiovascular Care Science With Treatment Recommendations Jeffrey M. Perlman, Jonathan Wyllie, John Kattwinkel, Dianne L. Atkins, Leon Chameides, Jay P. Goldsmith, Ruth Guinsburg, Mary Fran Hazinski, Colin Morley, Sam Richmond, Wendy M. Simon, Nalini Singhal, Edgardo Szyld, Masanori Tamura, Sithembiso Velaphi Neonatal Resuscitation Chapter Collaborators. Circulation 2010;122:S516-S538.

Part 11: Neonatal resuscitation 2010 International Consensus on Cardiopulmonary Resuscitation and Emergency Cardiovascular Care Science with Treatment Recommendations Jonathan Wyllie (Co-chair)*,1, Jeffrey M. Perlman (Co-chair)1, John Kattwinkel, Dianne L. Atkins, Leon Chameides, Jay P. Goldsmith, Ruth Guinsburg, Mary Fran Hazinski, Colin Morley, Sam Richmond, Wendy M. Simon, Nalini Singhal, Edgardo Szyld, Masanori Tamura, Sithembiso Velaphi Neonatal Resuscitation Chapter Collaborators. Resuscitation 2010; 81S: e260-e287.

European Resuscitation Council Guidelines for Resuscitation 2010 Section 7 Richmond S, Wyllie J. Resuscitation of babies at birth. Resuscitation 2010;81:1389-1399.

Ethical Considerations in Paediatric and Neonatal Life Support

CHAPTER 13

Learning outcomes

To understand:

- The legal and ethical implications of 'duty of care' with regard to paediatric resuscitation
- The indications for not starting resuscitation and the implications of this decision
- The considerations in the decision to stop a resuscitation attempt

Ethical concepts and principles

Ethics is the field of study that attempts to understand human actions in a moral sense. Medical ethics is the study of the application of moral principles that guide the behaviour of healthcare professionals. Ethical principles are not immutable; they change with the times and vary according to the social and cultural characteristics of human groups.

In the past, the ethics of medical practice have been guided by the Hippocratic principle 'Do good and avoid harm' without any recognition of the patient's opinion. Now, the central role of the patient (or parents/guardians in the case of a child) in the decision-making process is recognised. In the current approach to medical ethics, four guiding principles are considered:

- Autonomy
- Beneficence
- Justice
- Non-maleficence

Autonomy

The person who must make the final decisions about procedures and treatments is the adequately informed, competent patient. This principle requires that all healthcare professionals support the active participation of the patient in his treatment and decision-making. In paediatrics, it is fundamental to ensure that the parents/guardians have been correctly informed and that they fully understand the clinical situation, the treatment plan and alternatives before making a treatment decision. If the patient is not competent, because of age or disturbance of mental capability, the parents/guardians must make the decision on his behalf. The patient has a right to confidentiality: the doctor must inform only the patient and those individuals he wishes to be informed. The only exception to this is in the event of serious criminal actions where not informing a relevant authority would seriously jeopardise public welfare.

Competence

There may be occasions where a parent is absent and a condition is not life-threatening so professionals feel they cannot treat without permission but there is a degree of urgency. It may be the parental young person can give consent to treatment without the parent's consent, even if under 16 years. The criteria which should be followed are commonly known as the Fraser guidelines to determine if the young person under 16 years can give consent (having arisen in the area of contraception) but the Mental Health capacity Act 2005 covers the issues of children's consent in detail. All children aged 16 years and over are considered to have the capacity to consent to treatment unless there is evidence to the contrary.

The young person must understand the advice and have sufficient maturity to understand what is involved. The child must be able to retain the information and comprehend the nature, purpose and consequences of the treatment (or lack of it), and be able to communicate their decision. An example might include a limb-threatening rather than life threatening injury in a young teenager. The clinician must acknowledge that without the treatment, the young person's physical health may be at risk.

There may be occasions where the clinician disagrees with the parents. In a life threatening situation the clinician may act in the best interests of the child. If there is time the case can go to court for a judicial decision. In this instance, it is advisable that the clinician contact his defence organisation.

If a competent child is refusing treatment then those with parental responsibility can consent to treatment if this is in the child's best interests.

Beneficence

All medical acts must be guided by the goal of achieving good for the patient. This principle mandates that the patient is offered all available diagnostic procedures and potentially beneficial therapies.

Justice

It is mandatory to offer the same quality of care and support to all patients, without discrimination based on sex, race, religion or socioeconomics, and to guarantee equal opportunities and a rational distribution of resources. In addition, medical practice must conform to civilian and criminal law.

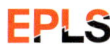

Non-maleficence

The actions of healthcare professionals must not cause harm. Treatments that are harmful must be avoided. The balance between risks and benefits of a proposed treatment for a patient must be evaluated carefully. Only treatments that have demonstrated efficacy should be used.

Ethical aspects of paediatric life support

Cardiorespiratory arrest and other clinical emergencies can be unpredictable. There may not be the opportunity to discuss treatment options with the child and/or parents/guardian before the event. In these circumstances, the principle of a child's autonomy is difficult to apply and healthcare professionals must make the decisions about resuscitation. In these situations, consent for life saving interventions is presumed.

For children, information must be given to the parents/guardians, unless the nature of the emergency does not allow this. If the parents/guardians are present, they can be given information as the resuscitation takes place; if they are not, the circumstances must be carefully documented in the child's medical records. In some cases, there may be conflicts of interest between parents, or they may refuse appropriate and effective treatment because of religious or other beliefs. If this occurs, the doctor must make a decision that protects the best interests of the child and he should request legal advice. Carefully detailed documentation including the reasons for the decision is vital.

Ethics and cardiorespiratory resuscitation

When to start resuscitation

Life support should be started in the following circumstances:

- Sudden and unexpected cardiorespiratory arrest.
- Recent cardiorespiratory arrest. However, if the delay in initiating resuscitation following cardiorespiratory arrest is more than 30 minutes, or if there are signs of established biological death, life support should not be started (with the exception of drowning and/or hypothermia).
- Potentially reversible cardiorespiratory arrest.
- Non-terminal illness. Resuscitation is not indicated if the cardiorespiratory arrest is the final natural end event in a process of dying after all available treatment options have been exhausted. The right to die with suitable dignity must be respected.
- A 'Do not attempt resuscitation (DNAR)' order does not exist.
- There is no risk to the rescuer.

If in doubt, resuscitate!

When to stop resuscitation

Resuscitation should be terminated when:

- There are signs of established biological death.
- The rescuer is too exhausted to continue or is in danger.
- Other victims who have a greater chance of survival require simultaneous life support but there are insufficient numbers of people to carry out resuscitation.
- A DNAR order exists.
- Life support has been continued for at least 20 minutes without evidence of a return of spontaneous circulation.

However, resuscitation should be continued:

- in hypothermic children
- in cases of poisoning
- in persistent ventricular fibrillation
- when cardiorespiratory arrest occurs in children with invasive monitoring in place (whereby coronary perfusion pressure can be continuously assessed so ensuring that an adequate cardiac output can be generated to perfuse vital organs)
- when the team considers (based on specific circumstances) that resuscitation efforts must be maintained

In newborn babies, after 10 minutes of optimal resuscitation, discontinuation may be justified if there are no signs of life.

Organ donation

International consensus is that brain stem death is equivalent to the death of the person. When brain stem death has occurred, the only rationale for maintaining cardiorespiratory function is to allow further investigations for organ donation. In these circumstances, if cardiac activity stops, resuscitation would be inappropriate.

Donation of an organ should be requested in the event of brain stem death, or for cardiac valve donation in the event of cardiac death. The approach to the family of the potential organ donor must be sensitive and respectful. Frequently this request is accepted, usually 'to help other children'. The donation should not impair the bereavement process of the child's family. Sometimes parents change their 'mind' many hours after a child's death and it is worth remembering some organs may still be useful such as corneas. Seek specialist advice as soon as possible.

Contraindications to organ donation are:

- Intravenous drug addiction
- Specific infections
- Metabolic diseases
- Cancers, except for certain non-metastatic brain tumours

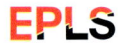

Do not attempt resuscitation order

A DNAR order requires the following to be considered:

- Anticipation of cardiorespiratory arrest. The order must be made prior to arrest, with agreement between the doctors in charge, all other healthcare professionals and the family
- Prognosis and expectation of quality of life
- Informed consent must be obtained, which takes into account ethical conditions and requirements

The DNAR order must be:

- In writing and included in the patient's medical notes
- Compatible with palliative care
- Regularly reviewed and can be revoked at any time

Presence of parents during resuscitation

Parents of children suffering from chronic diseases may be used to assisting with medical procedures and often are present during the resuscitation of their children.

The majority of parents would like to be present during resuscitation. Parents witnessing their child's resuscitation can see that everything possible has been attempted.

Families who are present at their child's death show less anxiety and depression, better adjustment and an improved grieving process when assessed several months later.

The opportunity to be present during resuscitation should be offered to parents. If they decide to stay, a dedicated member of the team must be assigned to explain the process to them in an empathetic manner, thereby ensuring that the parents do not interfere with resuscitation. When appropriate, physical contact with the child should be allowed and, wherever possible, the parents should be permitted to be with their dying child in the final moments.

The resuscitation team leader will decide when to stop resuscitation. This must be expressed to the parents with sensitivity and understanding.

Informing parents

When a child dies, it is the resuscitation team leader's duty to inform the parents. This is always a difficult task, particularly if the parents were not present at the resuscitation.

The following principles may ease the process:

- Select an appropriate environment (with assured privacy)
- Establish with certainty who the family members are, and their relationship to the child
- Explain with clarity that their child is dead (use the word "dead" specifically). Information should be given with empathy, compassion and sympathy. The details of the circumstances should be given clearly. Use the child's first name
- Encourage the parents to see and stay with their child. They should be encouraged to touch and hold their child
- The medical attitude must be professional, with a simple and clear explanation of the facts, but at the same time it should be compassionate and the emotional needs of the parents must be recognised
- Explain the necessity (if applicable) of a post-mortem examination, particularly in cases of sudden, unexplained or accidental death. Inform the parents that the police are routinely informed if the child's death fits these circumstances
- Permission for post-mortem studies should only be requested when the parents are in an acceptable emotional condition
- Ask the parents about any religious requirements
- Do not guess at the diagnosis but explain that the pathologist will try to ascertain the cause of death
- Make an appointment for further discussion and information

Verify

- Name and address of parents
- Date of birth of the deceased child
- Arrival time in the emergency department (if relevant)
- Time of death

Inform

- Paediatrician or general practitioner, giving the address where the parents are going and their contact details
- Health visitor for children < 5 years or school nurse for children > 5 years
- Social worker
- Persons that the parents wish to be informed
- Document this information in the child's notes and ensure their safe keeping

Chapter 13 Ethical Considerations in Paediatric and Neonatal Life Support

Key learning points

- Ethics attempts to understand human actions in a moral sense
- In current medical ethics, the four guiding principles are: autonomy, beneficence, non - maleficence and justice
- Information must be given to the child as appropriate and to the parents/guardians
- The majority of parents would like to be present during resuscitation.
- If the child dies, parents being present during resuscitation helps their grieving process

Further reading

Beckman AW, Sloan BK, Moore GP et al. Should parents be present during emergency department procedures on children, and who should make that decision? A survey of emergency physician and nurse attitudes. Acad Emerg Med 2002; 9: 154-8.

British Medical Association, Resuscitation Council (UK) and Royal College of Nursing. Decisions relating to cardiopulmonary resuscitation. 2007. www.resus.org.uk

Boie ET, Moore GP, Brummett C, Nelson DR. Do parents want to be present during invasive procedures performed on their children in the emergency department? A survey of 400 parents. Ann Emerg Med 1999; 34: 70-4.

Horisberger T, Fischer JE, Fanconi S. One-year survival and neurological outcome after pediatric cardiopulmonary resuscitation. Int Care Med 2002; 28: 365-8.

Powers KS, Rubenstein JS. Family presence during invasive procedures in the pediatric intensive care unit: a prospective study. Arch Pediatr Adoles Med 1999; 153: 955-8.

Meyers TA, Eichhorn DJ, Guzzetta CE et al. Family presence during invasive procedures and resuscitation. Am J Nurs 2000; 100: 32-42.

Sacchetti A, Lichenstein R, Carraccio CA, Harris RH. Family member presence during pediatric emergency department procedures. Pediatr Emerg Care 1996; 12: 268-71.

Robinson SM, Mackenzie-Ross S, Campbell Hewson GL, Egleston CV, Prevost AT. Psychological effect of witnessed resuscitation on bereaved relatives [comment]. Lancet 1998; 352: 614-7.

Sharp MC, Strauss RP, Lorch RC. Communicating medical bad news: parents' experiences and preferences. J Pediatr 1992; 121: 539-46.

Taylor N, Bonilla L, Silver P, Sagy M. Pediatric procedure: do parents want to be present? Crit Care Med 1996; 24: A131.

Tsai E. Should family members be present during cardiopulmonary resuscitation? N Engl J Med 2002; 346: 1019-21.

Woolley H, Stein A, Forest GC et al. Imparting the diagnosis of life threatening illness in children. BMJ 1989; 298: 1623-6.

Youngblut JM, Shiao SYP. Child and family reactions during and after pediatric ICU hospitalization: a pilot study. Heart Lung 1993; 22: 46-54.

I. Barata, J. LaMantia, D. Riccardi, et al: A Prospective Study of Emergency Medicine Residents' Attitudes toward Family Presence during Pediatric Procedures. . The Internet Journal of Emergency Medicine. 2007 Volume 3 Number 2.

L.Nibert, D.Ondrejka Family presence during pediatric resuscitation: An integrative review for evidence-based practice Journal of Pediatric Nursing 2005, Volume 20, Issue 2, Pages 145-147.

http://www.dca.gov.uk/menincap/legis.htm.

Human Factors and Quality in Resuscitation

CHAPTER 14

Learning outcomes

To understand:

▶ The role of human factors in resuscitation

▶ The roles of team leader and team member

▶ How to use structured communication tools such as SBAR and RSVP

Human factors

Paediatric resuscitation is stressful and sometimes highly time critical. To maximise the best care for the patient, it is important to reflect on and scrutinise every aspect of the resuscitation. This includes how it was conducted. Traditionally advanced life support courses have focused on the skills and knowledge required to deliver optimal care, but they have not considered the role of teams and their leadership. The medical fraternity has notably lagged behind organisations in considering how to manage crisis situations, for example, the world of aviation from which much may be learnt. This chapter considers those team roles and how teams are best led.

Critical decision making in a tense environment depends on many non-technical skills comprising team leadership, situational awareness, team membership, task distribution and above all communication amongst team members; these processes make up the 'Human factors'.

The resuscitation team is only as good as the weakest link and there is clear evidence from simulation in anaesthesia and neonatal courses that it is possible and practical to teach 'Crisis resource management' or 'Human factors'.

Deficiencies in the requisite non-technical skills are a common cause of adverse incidents. Analysis of adverse incidents in anaesthesia showed that in up to 80% of cases, there were failures in non-technical skills such as communication, checking drug doses, planning and team organisation, rather than equipment failure or lack of knowledge. As a result, the Anaesthetic Crisis Resource Management course was developed in America, followed by the Anaesthetists Non-Technical Skills (ANTS) system, pioneered by a team of anaesthetists and psychologists in Scotland (www.abdn.ac.uk/iprc/ants). The principles used to promote good non-technical skills in the UK Resuscitation courses are based on the principles of ANTS:

- Situational awareness
- Decision making
- Team working, including team leadership
- Task management

Situational awareness

This can be described as an individual's awareness of the environment at any one moment in a crisis and their ability to respond. How they react may impact on future events, this becomes particularly important when many events are happening simultaneously e.g. at a cardiorespiratory arrest. A lot of information input with poor situational awareness may result in the leader making poor decisions with serious consequences. At a cardiorespiratory arrest, all those participating will have varying degrees of situational awareness. In a well-functioning team, all members will have a common understanding of current events, or shared situational awareness. It is important that only the relevant information is shared otherwise there is too much distraction or background noise which may be irrelevant to the patient's immediate requirements.

Important situational awareness factors include:

- consideration of the location of the arrest, which can give clues to the cause;
- obtaining information from staff about the events leading up to the arrest;
- confirmation of the diagnosis;
- noting of actions already initiated e.g. chest compressions;
- checking that a monitor been attached and interpreting what it shows;
- communicating with the team, gathering information;
- implementing any immediate necessary action;
- consideration of the likely impact of interventions;
- determining the immediate needs.

Decision making

This is process of choosing a specific course of action from several alternatives. At a cardiorespiratory arrest, decision making usually falls to the most senior clinician present (e.g. nurse, junior doctor). This person will need to take on a leadership role before the resuscitation team arrives. The leader will assimilate information from those present and from personal observation and will use this to determine appropriate interventions. Typical decisions made include:

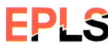

- confirmation of cardiorespiratory arrest;
- calling the resuscitation team;
- starting CPR;
- attaching a defibrillator and delivering a shock.

Once a decision has been made, clear unambiguous communication is essential to ensure that it is implemented. For example when a nurse finding a patient asks her colleague to call the resuscitation team – " John, this child is in cardiorespiratory arrest, please can you dial 2222 and call the resuscitation team and come back when you have done this".

Team working, including team leadership

Team leadership can be taught, observed and practised. Team membership can be improved by rehearsal, reflection and coaching producing effective teams which lead them to perform well together. By the end of the course, the candidate should understand the importance of the roles, both as a team leader and a team member.

Team leadership

The management of a sick child requires a team leader who provides guidance, direction and instruction to the team members. Team leaders lead by example and integrity, and need experience, not simply seniority. Team leadership is achieved as a process, thereby it can become available to everyone with training and it is not restricted to those with leadership traits. There are several attributes recognisable in good team leaders:

- Team leader knows everyone in the team by name and knows their capability.
- Accepts the leadership role.
- Is able to delegate tasks appropriately.
- Is knowledgeable and has sufficient credibility to influence the team through role modelling and professionalism.
- Remains calm and keeps everyone focused and controls distractions.
- Is a good communicator – not just good at giving instructions, also a good listener and decisive in action.
- Is assertive and authoritative when appropriate.
- Shows tolerance towards hesitancy or nervousness in the emergency setting, showing empathy towards the whole team
- Has good situational awareness: the ability to monitor the situation continuously, maintaining an up-to-date overview, as well as listening and deciding on a course of action.

During a cardiorespiratory arrest, the role of team leader is not always immediately obvious. The leader should state early on that they are assuming the role of team leader.

Specifically, the leader should:

- Allocate roles and tasks according to the strengths of team members and be specific.
- Follow current resuscitation guidelines or explain the reasoning for any significant deviation from standard protocols.
- If they are unsure, he or she should consult with the team or call for senior advice and assistance if appropriate.
- Allow the team some autonomy if their skills are adequate. This avoids several people or nobody attempting the task!
- Use the two-minute periods of chest compressions to plan tasks and safety aspects of the resuscitation attempt with the team.
- At the end of the resuscitation attempt, thank the team and ensure that staff and relatives are being supported. Complete all documentation and ensure an adequate handover.
- If a case is particularly complex it may be necessary for the leadership style to change from facilitative to directive in order to drive the speed of treatment in the time critical situation.

A doctor who is likely to lead a team should consider refreshing themselves with regard to:

- Staff on the shift
- Current guidelines
- Availability of sources of information whilst on duty
- Familiarise themselves with local equipment such as the defibrillator, type of intra-osseous needles/EZ-IO.
- Consider rehearsing scenarios either alone or with colleagues. For example, rehearsal of exercises such as "what if such and such a patient presents" followed by the clinician then detailing the patient's management has been shown to reduce stress and improve their performance.
- Consider their own strategies for stress reduction, how will they manage if a situation escalates?

Team membership

The resuscitation team may take the form of a traditional cardiac arrest team, which is called only when cardiorespiratory arrest is recognised. Alternatively, hospitals may have strategies to recognise sick children at risk of cardiorespiratory arrest and to summon a team (e.g. medical emergency team) before cardiorespiratory arrest occurs. The term 'resuscitation team' reflects the range of response teams. As the team may change daily or more frequently, as shift pattern working is introduced, members may not know each other or the skill mix of the team members. The team should therefore meet at the beginning of their period on duty to:

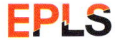

- Introduce themselves to each other; communication is easier and more effective if people can be referred to by their name.

- Identify everyone's skills and experience.

- Allocate the team leader role. Skill and experience should take precedence over seniority.

- Allocate responsibilities; if key skills are lacking, e.g. nobody skilled in tracheal intubation, work out how this deficit can be managed.

- Review any patients who have been identified as 'at risk' during the previous duty period.

Finally, every effort should be made to enable the team members to meet at the end of their duty to debrief (Figure 14.1), e.g. to discuss what went well and what could be improved. It may also be possible to carry out a formal handover to the incoming team.

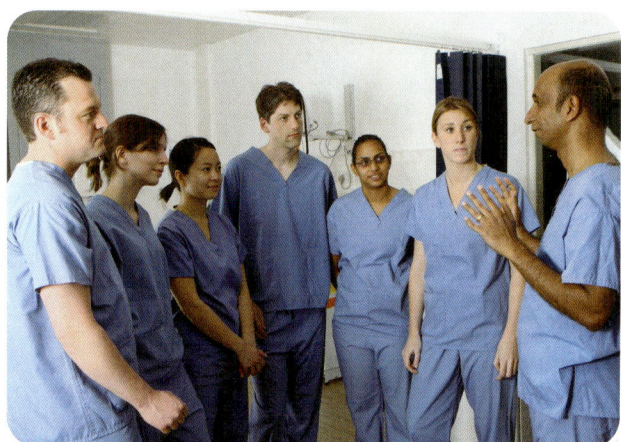

Figure 14.1 Team debrief

Teamwork is one of the most important non-technical skills that contribute to successful management of critical situations. A team is a group of individuals working together with a common goal or purpose. In a team, the members usually have complementary skills and, through coordination of effort, work synergistically. Teams work best when everyone knows each other's name, when they are doing something they perceive to be important, and when their role is within their experience and competence. Optimal team function mandates a team leader. There are several characteristics of a good resuscitation team member:

- Competence – has the skills required at a cardiorespiratory arrest and performs them to the best of their ability.

- Commitment – strives to achieve the best outcome for the patient.

- Communicates – openly, indicating their findings and actions taken, and be prepared to raise concerns about clinical or safety issues, but also by listening to briefings and instructions from the team leader.

- Supportive and facilitative – allows others to achieve their best.

- Accountable – for their own and the team's actions and to be prepared to admit when help is needed.

- Creative – suggests different ways of interpreting the situation.

- Participates in providing feedback.

Task management

The many decisions to be made usually fall to the team leader. The leader will assimilate information from the team members and from personal observation, and will use this to determine appropriate interventions. Typical decisions made include:

- diagnosis of the cardiorespiratory arrest rhythm;

- choice of shock energy to be used for defibrillation;

- likely reversible causes of the cardiorespiratory arrest;

- how long to continue resuscitation.

Once a decision has been made, clear unambiguous communication with the team members is essential to ensure that it is implemented.

During the resuscitation, there are numerous tasks to be carried out by the team members, either sequentially or simultaneously. The coordination and control, or management of these tasks is the responsibility of the team leader. They include:

- Planning, where appropriate and briefing the team, prior to the arrival of the patient.

- Being inclusive of team members.

- Being prepared for both the expected and the unexpected.

- Identification of resources required – ensure that equipment is checked and specifics organised and delegated.

- Prioritising actions of the team.

- Watching out for fatigue, stress and distress amongst the team.

- Managing conflict.

- Communicating with relatives.

- Communicating with experts for safe handover both by telephone and in person.

- Debriefing the team.

- Reporting untoward incidents, particularly equipment or system failures (see below).

- Participation in audit.

Communication

Communication problems are a factor in up to 80% of adverse incidents or near miss reports in hospitals.

Communication is vital in every stage of managing a sick child, in summoning help, in preparing for the resuscitation, during the resuscitation and in organising the post resuscitation care. The use of the SBAR (Situation-Background-Assessment-Recommendation) or RSVP (Reason, Story, Vital signs, Plan) tool enables effective, timely communication between individuals from different clinical backgrounds and hierarchies.

Initial stage

When individuals are faced with a deteriorating patient it is beneficial if they can request help by presenting a succinct summary to a senior colleague. The SBAR and RSVP systems are validated tools for this purpose (Table 14.1).

Preparation

The team leader should learn people's names and abilities, this helps create the initial team. Good communication with the team members results in the appropriate task allocation and identifies if further senior help is required. If there are sufficient members, one person may be delegated to managing the airway, another the breathing, and another the circulation. The team leader can explain that he will ask in turn how the airway, breathing and circulation are, in order, and to ensure that this order of priority of treatment is followed should any problems be found. The team leader should explain that he will ask for reassessment of the ABCDE, to see the effects of any interventions that have been carried out.

Preparation can made if there is time by writing up predicted requirements, if the age or weight of the child is known. Frequently, a pre-alert for a child arriving by ambulance of his age allows for estimation of equipment, fluid and drugs prior to his arrival.

Management of the resuscitation

During the resuscitation phase, clear commands addressed directly to individuals keeps a team focused and a team leader should use closed loop techniques to ensure a task has been performed e.g. "bloods taken, including gases and cross match 4 units packed cells".

It may be helpful to ask in turn the findings of the person dealing with the Airway, then Breathing and then the Circulation, addressing any problems that are found as they are identified.

Post resuscitation care

Resuscitation does not stop with ROSC. Handing the patient over to another colleague, or department or to a different hospital all requires good communication and the SBAR or RSVP tool can provide a framework for information sharing at this stage.

High quality care

The Institute of Medicine defines that quality care is safe, effective, patient-centred, timely, efficient and equitable. Hospitals, resuscitation teams and EPLS providers should ensure they deliver these aspects of quality to improve the care of the deteriorating patient and patients in cardiorespiratory arrest. Two aspects of this are safety incident reporting (also called adverse or critical incident reporting) and collecting good quality data.

Safety incident reporting

In England and Wales, hospitals can report patient safety incidents to the National Patient Safety Agency (NPSA) National Reporting and Learning System (NRLS) (http://www.nrls.npsa.nhs.uk/report-a-patient-safety-incident/). A patient safety incident is defined as 'any unintended or unexpected incident that could have harmed or did lead to harm for one or more patients being cared for by the National Health Service (NHS). Previous reviews of this database have identified patient safety incidents associated with airway devices in critical care units and led to recommendations to improve safety. A review of NPSA safety incidents relating to cardiorespiratory arrest and patient deterioration by the Resuscitation Council (UK) shows that the most common reported incidents are associated with equipment problems, communication, delays in the resuscitation team attending and failure to escalate treatment.

Audit and outcome after cardiac arrest

Most modern defibrillators allow the cardiorespiratory arrest management to be downloaded with a time-line of different rhythms and actions taken in terms of defibrillation and cardioversion. Locally, this useful information can help teams by reflection and feedback on performance especially in terms of adherence to resuscitation guidelines, the percentage of time CPR has been performed and "hands-off" time.

National audit of the processes and outcomes provides information about whether interventions and changes made to resuscitation guidelines improve patient care. There is lack of uniformity in reporting both the process and results of resuscitation attempts; for example, the definition of survival is reported variously as return of spontaneous circulation, or survival at 5 min, 1 h, 24 h, or to discharge from hospital. The lack of uniformity in cardiorespiratory arrest reporting makes it difficult to evaluate the impact on survival of individual factors, such as new drugs or techniques.

New interventions that improve survival rate only slightly are important because of the many victims of cardiorespiratory arrest each year. Local hospitals or healthcare systems are unlikely to have sufficient patients to identify these effects or eliminate confounders. One way around this dilemma is by adopting uniform definitions and collecting standardised data on both the process and outcome of resuscitation on many patients in multiple centres. Changes in the resuscitation process can then be introduced and evaluated using a

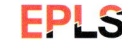

SBAR	RSVP	Content	Example

SITUATION	**R**EASON	• Introduce yourself and check you are speaking to the correct person
		• Identify the patient you are calling about (who and where)
		• Say what you think the current problem is, or appears to be
		• State what you need advice about
		• Useful phrases:
		  - The problem appears to be cardiac/respiratory/neurological/sepsis
		  - I'm not sure what the problem is but the patient is deteriorating
		  - The patient is unstable, getting worse and I need help
			• Hi, I'm Dr Smith the paediatric F2
			• I am calling about Sam Brown on the paediatric ward who I think has a severe pneumonia and is septic
			• He has an oxygen saturation of 90% despite high-flow oxygen and I am very worried about him

BACKGROUND	**S**TORY	• Background information about the patient • Reason for admission • Relevant past medical history	• He is 6 years old and previously fit and well • He has had fever and a cough for 2 days • He was admitted yesterday
ASSESSMENT	**V**ITAL SIGNS	• Include specific observations and vital sign values based on ABCDE approach • Airway • Breathing • Circulation • Disability • Exposure • The early warning score is…	• He looks very unwell and is tiring • Airway – he can say a few words • Breathing – his respiratory rate is 34, he has widespread wheeze in both lung fields and has bronchial breathing on the left side. His oxygen saturation is 90% on high-flow oxygen. I am getting a blood gas and chest X-ray • Circulation – his pulse is 180, his blood pressure is 90/60 • Disability – he is drowsy and is clinging onto his mum • Exposure – he has no rashes

RECOMMENDATION	**P**LAN	• State explicitly what you want the person you are calling to do
		• What by when?
		• Useful phrases:
		  - I am going to start the following treatment; is there anything else you can suggest?
		  - I am going to do the following investigations; is there anything else you can suggest?
		  - If they do not improve; when would you like to be called?
		  - I don't think I can do any more; I would like you to see the patient urgently
			• He is only on oral antibiotics so I am starting an IV
			• I need help – please can you come and see him straight away?

Table 14.1 SBAR and RSVP communication tools

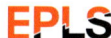

reliable measure of outcome. This methodology enables drugs and techniques developed in experimental studies to be evaluated reliably in the clinical setting.

In the UK, the National Cardiac Arrest Audit (NCAA) is an ongoing, national, comparative outcome audit of in-hospital cardiac arrests. It is a joint initiative between the Resuscitation Council (UK) and the Intensive Care National Audit & Research Centre (ICNARC) and is open to all acute hospitals in the UK and Ireland. The audit monitors and reports on the incidence of, and outcome from, in-hospital cardiorespiratory arrest in order to inform practice and policy. It aims to identify and foster improvements in the prevention, care delivery and outcomes from cardiorespiratory arrest. The initial scope of data collection is patients who meet all of the following criteria:

- Adults or children over 28 days of age
- Receive chest compressions and/or defibrillation
- Attended by the hospital-based resuscitation team (or equivalent) in response to a 2222 call.

Data are collected according to standardised definitions and entered onto the NCAA secure web-based system. Once data are validated, hospitals are provided with activity reports and comparative reports, allowing a comparison of to be made not only within, but also between, hospitals locally, nationally and internationally. Furthermore it also enables the effects of introducing changes to guidelines, new drugs, new techniques etc to be monitored that would not be possible on a hospital-by-hospital basis.

Key learning points

- **Human factors are important during resuscitation**
- **Use SBAR or RSVP for effective communication**
- **Report safety incidents and collect cardiac arrest data to help improve patient care**

Further reading

Flin R, O'Connor P, Crichton M. Safety at the Sharp End: a Guide to Non-Technical Skills. Aldershot: Ashgate, 2008.

Flin R, Patey R, Glavin R, Maran N. Anaesthetists' non-technical skills. Br J Anaesth 2010; 105: 38-44.

Acknowledgement

The Resuscitation Council (UK) would like to express its thanks to Professor Rhona Flin, University of Aberdeen, for permission to use of the Anaesthetists Non-Technical Skills (ANTS) system.

Appendix 1: Paediatric Emergency Drug Chart

	ADRENALINE	FLUID BOLUS	GLUCOSE	SODIUM BICARBONATE		TRACHEAL TUBE UNCUFFED	TRACHEAL TUBE CUFFED	DEFIBRILLATION
STRENGTH	1:10,000	0.9% Saline	10%	4.2%	8.4%			4 joules kg^{-1}
DOSE	10 mcg kg^{-1}	20 ml kg^{-1}	2 ml kg^{-1}	1 mmol kg^{-1}				Trans-thoracic
ROUTE	IV, IO	IV, IO	IV, IO	IV, IO, UVC	IV, IO			Monophasic or biphasic
NOTES		Consider warmed fluids	For known hypoglycaemia. Recheck glucose after dose				Monitor cuff pressure	
AGE / WEIGHT kg	ml	ml	ml	ml	ml	ID mm	ID mm	Manual
<1 month / 3.5	0.35	70	7	7	-	3.0	-	20
1 month / 4	0.4	80	8	8	-	3.0 - 3.5	3.0	20
3 months / 5	0.5	100	10	10	-	3.5	3.0	20
6 months / 7	0.7	140	14	-	7	3.5	3.0	30
1 year / 10	1.0	200	20	-	10	4.0	3.5	40
2 years / 12	1.2	240	24	-	12	4.5	4.0	50
3 years / 14	1.4	280	28	-	14	4.5 - 5.0	4.0 - 4.5	60
4 years / 16	1.6	320	32	-	16	5.0	4.5	60
5 years / 18	1.8	360	36	-	18	5.0 - 5.5	4.5 - 5.0	70
6 years / 20	2.0	400	40	-	20	5.5	5.0	80
7 years / 23	2.3	460	46	-	23	5.5 - 6.0	5.0 - 5.5	90
8 years / 26	2.6	520	52	-	26	-	6.0 - 6.5	100
10 years / 30	3.0	600	60	-	30	-	7.0	120
12 years / 38	3.8	760	76	-	38	-	7 - 7.5	150
Adolescent / >40kg	10	1000	80	-	50	-	7 - 8	As for adults

Cardioversion Synchronised Shock – 0.5-1.0 joules kg^{-1} escalating to 2.0 joules kg^{-1} if unsuccessful.
Amiodarone 5 mg kg^{-1} IV or IO bolus in arrest (0.1 ml kg^{-1} of 150 mg in 3 ml) after 3rd and 5th shocks. Flush line with 0.9% saline or 5% glucose.
Atropine 20 mcg kg^{-1}, minimum dose 100 mcg, maximum dose 600 mcg.
Calcium chloride 10% 0.2 ml kg^{-1} for hypocalcaemia / hyperkalaemia.
Lorazepam 100 mcg kg^{-1} IV or IO for treatment of seizures. Can be repeated after 10 minutes. Maximum single dose 4mg.
Naloxone Resuscitation dose for full reversal 100 mcg kg^{-1}. For partial reversal of opiate analgesia 10 mcg kg^{-1} boluses, titrated to effect.
Anaphylaxis Adrenaline 1:1000 **intramuscularly** (<6 yrs 150 mcg [0.15 ml], 6-12 yrs 300 mcg [0.3 ml], >12 yrs 500 mcg [0.5ml]) can be repeated after five minutes. **OR** titrate boluses of 1 mcg kg^{-1} IV **ONLY** if familiar with giving IV adrenaline.

Weights averaged on lean body mass from 50th centile weights for males and females. Drug doses based on Resuscitation Council (UK) Guidelines 2010 recommendations. Recommendations for tracheal tubes are based on full term neonates.
For newborns glucose at 2.5ml kg^{-1} is recommended.

EUROPEAN PAEDIATRIC LIFE SUPPORT

Appendix 1. Paediatric Emergency Drug Chart

Appendix 2. Pulse Oximetry and Oxygen Therapy

Introduction

Pulse oximetry is used to assess the patient's arterial oxygen saturation. Without pulse oximetry, you may not notice the patient has a decreased arterial oxygen saturation of haemoglobin (SaO_2) until the saturation is between 80-85%. Pulse oximetry is simple to use, relatively cheap, non-invasive and provides an immediate, objective measure of arterial blood oxygen saturation.

The pulse oximeter probe containing light-emitting diodes (LEDs) and a photoreceptor situated opposite, is placed across tissue, usually a finger or earlobe. Some of the light is transmitted through the tissues while some is absorbed. The ratio of transmitted to absorbed light is used to generate the peripheral arterial oxygen saturation (SpO_2) displayed as a digital reading, waveform, or both.

Most pulse oximeters have an audible tone related to the SpO_2, with a decreasing tone reflecting increasing hypoxaemia. The pulse rate is also usually displayed. A poor signal indicates a low blood pressure or poor tissue perfusion – reassess the patient.

Pulse oximeter readings must not be used in isolation: it is vital to interpret them in light of the clinical picture and alongside other investigations, and potential sources of error. Pulse oximetry provides only a measure of oxygen saturation, not content, and thus gives no indication of actual tissue oxygenation. Furthermore, it provides no information on adequacy of ventilation. A patient may be breathing inadequately and have a high carbon dioxide level despite a normal oxygen saturation. Arterial blood gases are needed in critically ill patients to assess oxygenation and ventilation.

Limitations

The relationship between oxygen saturation and arterial oxygen partial pressure (PaO_2) is demonstrated by the oxyhaemoglobin dissociation curve (Figure A.2). The sinusoid shape of the curve means that an initial decrease from a normal PaO_2 is not accompanied by a drop of similar magnitude in the oxygen saturation of the blood, and early hypoxaemia may be masked. At the point where the SpO_2 reaches 90-92%, the PaO_2 will have decreased to around 8 kPa. In other words, the partial pressure of oxygen in the arterial blood will have decreased by almost 50% despite a reduction in oxygen saturation of only 6-8%.

The output from a pulse oximeter relies on a comparison between current signal output and standardised reference data derived from healthy volunteers. Readings provided are thus limited by the scope of the population included in these studies, and become increasingly unreliable with increasing hypoxaemia. Below 70% the displayed values are highly unreliable.

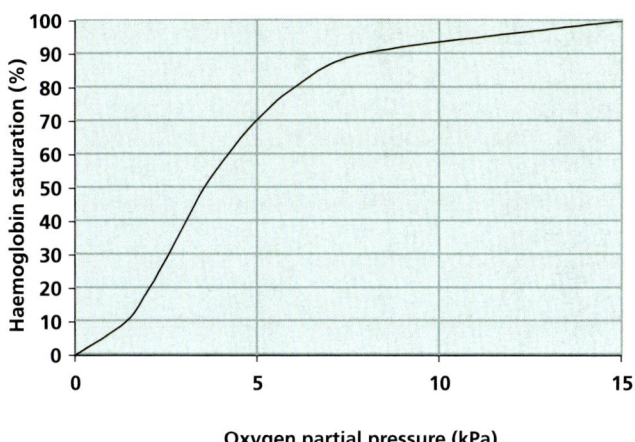

Figure A.2 Oxyhaemoglobin dissociation curve

There are several acknowledged sources of error with pulse oximetry:

- Presence of other haemoglobins: carboxyhaemoglobin (carbon monoxide poisoning) and methaemoglobin (congenital or acquired)
- Surgical and imaging dyes: methylene blue, indocyanine green and indigo carmine cause falsely low saturation readings
- Nail varnish (especially blue, black and green)
- High-ambient light levels (fluorescent and xenon lamps)
- Motion artefact
- Reduced pulse volume:
    - Hypotension
    - Low cardiac output
    - Vasoconstriction
    - Hypothermia

Pulse oximeters are not affected by:

- Anaemia (reduced haemoglobin concentration)
- Jaundice (hyperbilirubinaemia)
- Skin pigmentation

Pulse oximetry does not provide a reliable signal during CPR.

Appendix 2. Pulse Oximetry and Oxygen Therapy

Uses

Pulse oximetry has four main uses:

1. detection of/screening for hypoxaemia;
2. targeting oxygen therapy;
3. routine monitoring during anaesthesia;
4. diagnostic (e.g. sleep apnoea).

Targeted oxygen therapy

In critically ill patients, those presenting with acute hypoxaemia (initial SpO_2 <85%), or in the peri-arrest situation, give high-concentration oxygen immediately. Give this initially with an oxygen mask and reservoir ('non-rebreathing' mask) and an oxygen flow of 15 l min^{-1}. During cardiorespiratory arrest use 100% oxygen to maximise arterial oxygen content and delivery to the tissues.

Once return of spontaneous circulation has been achieved and the oxygen saturation of arterial blood can be monitored reliably, adjust the inspired oxygen concentration to maintain a SpO_2 of 94-98%. If pulse oximetry (with a reliable reading) is unavailable, continue oxygen via a reservoir mask until definitive monitoring or assessment of oxygenation is available. All critically ill patients will need arterial blood gas sampling and analysis as soon as possible. Evidence suggests both hypoxaemia and hyperoxaemia (PaO_2 > 20 kPa) in the post-resuscitation phase may lead to worse outcomes than those in whom normoxaemia is maintained.

Further reading

ILCOR Worksheet on oxygen administration
http://www.americanheart.org/presenter.jhtml?identifier=3065183.

O'Driscoll BR, Howard LS, Davison AG. BTS guideline for emergency oxygen use in adult patients. Thorax 2008;63 Suppl 6:vi1-68.

Appendix 3.
Asthma Algorithms

The two paediatric algorithms included in this appendix are reproduced from:

The British Guideline on the Management of Asthma
A national clinical guideline
Revised in 2009

Published by the British Thoracic Society and the Scottish Intercollegiate Guidelines Network.

© Scottish Intercollegiate Guidelines Network and British Thoracic Society

BTS/SIGN Guideline on the Management of Asthma, 2009
http://www.brit-thoracic.org.uk/clinical-information/asthma/asthma-guidelines.aspx

Appendix 3. Asthma Algorithms

MANAGEMENT OF ACUTE ASTHMA IN CHILDREN AGED OVER 2 YEARS

ACUTE SEVERE	LIFE THREATENING
SpO_2 <92% PEF 33-50% - Can't complete sentences in one breath or too breathless to talk or feed - Pulse >125 (>5 years) or >140 (2 to 5 years) - Respiration >30 breaths/min (>5 years) or >40 (2 to 5 years)	SpO_2 <92% PEF <33-50% best or predicted - Hypotension - Silent chest - Exhaustion - Cyanosis - Confusion - Poor respiratory effort - Coma

CRITERIA FOR ADMISSION

- ☑ β_2 agonists should be given as first line treatment. Increase β_2 agonist dose by two puffs every two minutes according to response up to ten puffs.

- ☑
  - Children with acute asthma in primary care who have not improved after receiving up to 10 puffs of β_2 agonist should be referred to hospital. Further doses of bronchodilator should be given as necessary whilst awaiting transfer
  - Treat children transported to hospital by ambulance with oxygen and nebulised β2 agonists during the journey.

- ☑ Paramedics attending to children with acute asthma should administer nebulised salbutamol driven by oxygen if symptoms are severe whilst transferring the child to the emergency department.

- ☑ Children with severe or life threatening asthma should be tranferred to hospital urgently.

- **B** Consider intensive inpatient treatment for children with SpO_2 <92% on air after initial bronchodilator treatment.

The following clinical signs should be recorded:
- **Pulse rate** - increasing tachycardia generally denotes worsening asthma; a fall in heart rate in life threatening asthma is a pre-terminal event
- **Respiratory rate and degree of breathlessness** - ie too breathless to complete sentences in one breath or to feed
- **Use of accessory muscles of respiration** - best noted by palpation of neck muscles
- **Amount of wheezing** - which might become biphasic or less apparent with increasing airways obstruction
- **Degree of agitation and conscious level** - always give calm reassurance

NB Clinical signs correlate poorly with the severity of airways obstruction. Some children with acute asthma do not appear distressed.

TREATMENT OF ACUTE ASTHMA

OXYGEN

- ☑ Children with life threatening asthma or SpO2 <94% should receive high flow oxygen via a tight fitting face mask or nasal cannula at sufficient flow rates to achieve normal saturations.

β2 AGONIST BRONCHODILATORS

- **A**
  - Inhaled β_2 agonists are the first line treatment for acute asthma
  - A pMDI + spacer is the preferred option in mild to moderate asthma.

- **B** Individualise drug dosing according to severity and adjust according to the patient's response.

- **B** Consider early addition of a single bolus dose of IV salbutamol (15 mcg/kg over 10 minutes) in severe cases where the patient has not responded to initial inhaled therapy.

- ☑ Discontinue long-acting β_2 agonists when short-acting β_2 agonists are required more often than four-hourly.

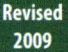

MANAGEMENT OF ACUTE ASTHMA IN CHILDREN AGED OVER 2 YEARS

STEROID THERAPY

A | Give prednisolone early in the treatment of acute asthma attacks.

☑
- Use a dose of 20 mg prednisolone for children aged 2 to 5 years and a dose of 30 - 40 mg for children >5 years. Those already receiving maintenance steroid tablets should receive 2 mg/kg prednisolone up to a maximum dose of 60 mg
- Repeat the dose of prednisolone in children who vomit and consider IV steroids
- Treatment for up to three days is usually sufficient, but the length of course should be tailored to the number of days necessary to bring about recovery. Weaning is unnecessary unless the course of steroids exceeds 14 days.

OTHER THERAPIES

A | If symptoms are refractory to initial β_2 agonist treatment, add ipratropium bromide (250 mcg/dose mixed with the nebulised β_2 agonist solution).

☑ | Repeated doses of ipratropium bromide should be given early to treat children poorly responsive to β_2 agonists.

A
C
- Aminophylline is not recommended in children with mild to moderate acute asthma
- Consider aminophylline in an HDU or PICU setting for children with severe or life threatening bronchospasm unresponsive to maximal doses of bronchodilators plus steroids.

☑ | Do not give antibiotics routinely in the management of acute childhood asthma.

MANAGEMENT OF ACUTE ASTHMA IN CHILDREN AGED UNDER 2 YEARS

- The assessment of acute asthma in early childhood can be difficult
- Intermittent wheezing attacks are usually due to viral infection and the response to asthma medication is inconsistent
- The differential diagnosis of symptoms includes:
    - aspiration pneumonitis
    - pneumonia
    - bronchiolitis
    - tracheomalacia
    - complications of underlying conditions such as congenital anomalies and cystic fibrosis
- Prematurity and low birth weight are risk factors for recurrent wheezing

TREATMENT OF ACUTE ASTHMA

β_2 AGONIST BRONCHODILATORS

B | Oral β_2 agonists are not recommended for acute asthma in infants.

A | For mild to moderate acute asthma, a pMDI+spacer is the optimal drug delivery device.

STEROID THERAPY

B | Consider steroid tablets in infants early in the management of moderate to severe episodes of acute asthma in the hospital setting.

☑ | Steroid tablet therapy (10 mg of soluble prednisolone for up to three days) is the preferred steroid preparation for use in this age group.

B | Consider inhaled ipratropium bromide in combination with an inhaled β_2 agonist for more severe symptoms.

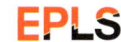

Appendix 3. Asthma Algorithms

Appendix 4. Useful Websites

www.resus.org.uk	Resuscitation Council UK
www.erc.edu	European Resuscitation Council
www.ilcor.org	International Liaison Committee on Resuscitation (ILCOR) – 2010 Consensus
www.bcs.com	British Cardiac Society
www.escardio.org	European Society of Cardiology
www.heart.org	American Heart Association
www.ics.ac.uk	Intensive Care Society
www.apagbi.org.uk	Association of Paediatric Anaesthetists of Great Britain and Ireland
www.bestbets.org	Best evidence topics in emergency medicine
www.rcpch.ac.uk	Royal College of Paediatrics and Child Health
www.library.nhs.uk	NHS Evidence
www.apem.me.uk	Association of Paediatric Emergency Medicine
www.stars.org.uk	Syncope Trust and Reflexic Anoxic Seizures
www.bnfc.org	British National Formulary for Children
www.trauma.org	Trauma Information Site
www.nice.org.uk	National Institute for Health and Clinical Excellence
www.sign.ac.uk	Scottish Intercollegiate Guidelines Network
www.brit-thoracic.org.uk	British Thoracic Society
www.hpa.org.uk	Health Protection Agency
www.uk-sands.org	Stillbirth and Neonatal Death Charity

NOTES

ET SIZE $\frac{AGE}{4} + 4$ Weight   Age + 4 × 2